GENITAL HERPES
MY FRIEND THE ENEMY

Edition 2022

"To Be, or Not to Be"
HERPES FREE

by REINHARD HERMES, MS

Copyright © 2022 Reinhard Hermes, MS
All Rights Reserved

No part of this book may be reproduced, scanned, or distributed in any form or by any electronic means, including information storage and retrieval systems, without the written consent from the author, except for the use of brief quotations in a book review. Otherwise, General, I mean, Genital Herpes Sputnik may infect you.

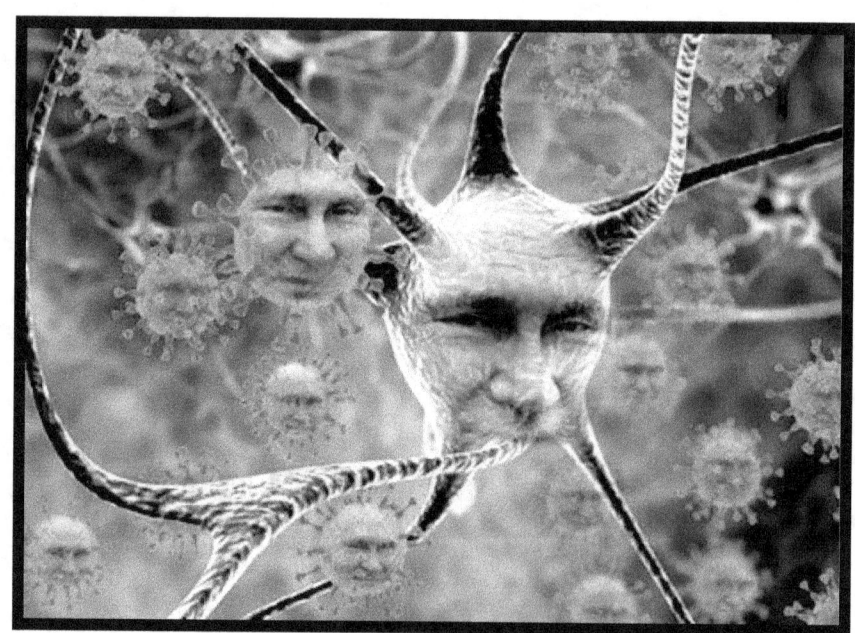

Table of Contents

TABLE OF CONTENTS III

DISCLAIMER VI

PREFACE VII

INTRODUCTION X

PART ONE: IN THE BEGINNING 1

CHAPTER 1: RX FOR HUMOR 2
    A. Herpes1 vs. Hermes1 3
    B. Berlin L.A. Express 4
    C. 80's Wannabees 4
    D. Stigma & Disclosure 6
    E. Double Edged Support 7
    F. Pregnancy 9
    G. Know Your Cause 10
    H. Grim Side Effects 12
    I. The ol' Mule 13

CHAPTER 2: LIVING SICK, DYING YOUNG 15
    A. Negativity Bias. 16
    B. Chronic Outbreaks 17
    C. Health Crisis 18
    D. Orthodox or Alternative 19
    E. Birth of Herpes 21
    F. Jokes, Scams, and Myths 22
    G. Out of Love 24

PART TWO: HERPES LIFE CYCLE 32

CHAPTER 3: HERPES 33
    A. Revenge of the Hippies 35
    B. Cold Sores (HSV-1) 39
    C. Other Oral Infections 40
    D. Genital Herpes (HSV-2) 41
    E. Shingles 45
    F. Getting Tested 45
    G. Not Getting Infected 47
    H. Isolation Viral 48

CHAPTER 4: ECZEMA HERPETICUM ... 51

CHAPTER 5: ORTHODOX MEDICINE ... 55
- A. First Outbreak ... 56
- B. Antiviral Medications ... 59
- C. Every Day or As Needed ... 61
- D. Risks & Side Effects ... 62
- E. Strategies on the Horizon ... 63
- F. Leaky Gut ... 65

CHAPTER 6: WHITE-COAT HUNTERS ... 67
- A. Bullets vs. Band-Aids ... 68
- B. God Heals, Drugs Mask & Parade ... 69

PART THREE: HEALING THE BODY ... 71

CHAPTER 7: PILLARS OF HEALTH ... 72
- A. Four Pillars of Health ... 73
- B. Three Undervalued Pillars ... 74
- C. The Immune System ... 80
- D. Sixteen Symptoms ... 83
- E. Hormones and Herpes ... 84

CHAPTER 8: START TODAY ... 89
- A. Forks and Knives ... 90
- B. Healthy Food Choices ... 91
- C. Nutrition for Herpes ... 93
- D. Chlorine-Fluoride-Bromine ... 96
- E. Hacking the Mind ... 97

CHAPTER 9: LIFESTYLE INFLUENCES ... 102
- A. Risk Factors ... 102
- B. Sleep ... 103
- C. Stress ... 105
- D. Exercise ... 106
- E. Alcohol ... 107

CHAPTER 10: PROTOCOLS ... 108
- A. The Beck Protocol ... 109
- B. Colloidal Silver ... 117
- C. Cell Salts ... 121
- D. DMSO ... 125
- E. High-Dose Vitamin C ... 127

   F. Low Dose Naltrexone (LDN) 132
   G. Chlorine Dioxide or **MMS1** 133
   H. Proteolytic Enzymes 142

CHAPTER 11: SUPPLEMENTS 145
   A. Immune Support Vitamins 146
   B. Immune Balancing 151
   C. Antiviral Supplements 154
   D. Topical Antivirals 166

PART FOUR: HEALING THE MIND 169

CHAPTER 12: PSYCHOLOGY OF HEALTH 170
   A. EFT Tapping 170
   B. Dapper Tappers 175
   C. Herpes Tapping Script 176
   D. Medication to Meditation 177
   E. Inside Outside Review 182

PART FIVE: HERMES PROTOCOL 183

CHAPTER 13: DAY-TO-DAY 187
   A. Morning 188
   B. Lunch 192
   C. Dinner & Evenings 193
   D. Detoxification 195

CHAPTER 14: IN CLOSING 202
   A. Peace for Happiness 203
   B. Fear to Confidence 206

DEDICATION 208

ABOUT THE AUTHOR 208

UNIFORM RESOURCE LOCATORS URLS 209

Disclaimer

The information in this book is my personal accounting and history with Genital Herpes. It is not meant to be used, and neither should be utilized to diagnose or treat any medical condition. Please consult your personal physician for diagnosis and/or treatment for any medical problem.

The author is not responsible or liable for any specific health or medical requirements that may arise from any treatment, action, application, or preparation, to any person reading or following the information as outlined in this book. This is strictly my subjective history, and any references provided are for informational purposes only and do not endorse any website or other sources listed in this book.

Also, please be aware that the websites and links in this book may change. They often do. In addition, the author does not have any financial relationship with any source listed in this book. Any names, situations, or details of information are either the authors or changed to protect the privacy of individuals. Thank you for your understanding in these matters.

Preface

Officer Brezhnev: across a barren Mojave wasteland, a dust-laden Santa Ana wind gathered storm and swooshed across Saddleback Mountain into Orange County's snarled Monday morning commute. Southern California's drought-stricken heat is a constant blustery threat to unleash a devastating firestorm without the thinnest provocation. The Mama & the Papas *California Dreamin'* often turned into a *Golden State Firemare*.

But this morning's breeze was of little concern to the prowess of the Jaguar bounding through Laguna Canyon. If traffic held, John Wayne Airport was only a 15-minute leap, and the 12-cylinder convertible would still have time to quaff down its prey, an Espresso-Macchiato. He glanced at the speedometer and leaned the Jag deep into the on-ramp. *"Oh, crap."* It didn't seem like he was doing ninety (90-mph). He took his foot off the accelerator and prepared to merge into a sluggish, grazing herd of European imports moseying down the 405 freeway.

The sun blinded his daydream. Adjusting his visor, crimson bright flashes appeared in his vision. *"Got to get some new Ray-Bans,"* he thought. Then without warning, the kaleidoscope of colors burst into a distressed wailing siren, and a galactic Star Wars storm-trooper appeared in his mirror, signaling the hunted to let go of his big-game fantasy and pull over. The BMW motorcycle lurched, leaned low against the wind, lights, sirens blaring. His Jaguar had turned into a pussycat. No match for a roaring lionhearted **California Highway Patrol (CHP)** officer.

The herd let out a *"I'm glad it's you"* exhaust, as the CHP officer motioned the Jag to pull over. The officer dismounted and took a minute to catch his breath, then approached a bit unsteady, while he adjusted his vest and chiseled upside-down demeanor. His expression said this was not going to be a palsy-walsy *Support-Your-Local-Police* bumper sticker chit-chat, or a name-dropping, banter about *"my Uncle Reinecke, the Lt. Governor."* Taking his helmet off, the officer wiped his Brezhnev eyebrows and let out a visible sigh. It was a time before COVID and facemasks.

"License and registration, please!"

He fumbled through the glove compartment and pried his driver's license from an imprisoned plastic sheath and handed it along with the registration to the officer.

"Do you know how fast you were going?"

"Yes, Officer… about 75 or 80."

"I clocked you at a 100. And with the wind, you put my life at risk."

"Oh crap." The Sirocco Triangle effect was at work with the officer's perception. He started to object but the officer withdrew his hand from the Glock as if directing traffic and said,

"Explain it to the judge and stay in your car."

"I'm in deep do-do," he thought and observed the customary warrant check in the rear-view mirror. The officer came back, looking pleased.

"I'm not going to write you up for doing a 100 and reckless driving. Then I'd have to arrest you and spend half my day doing paperwork. Verify your full name and is this still your current address?"

"Thank you, Officer… thank you… yes, yes… Reinhard Hermes, and yes, it is." He handed me the tablet, along with a routine guiltless admissions monologue and a smirking smile, then asked me to sign a 90 MPH speeding ticket, promising to appear or pay the fine.

"Officer, you're smiling. Is there something I missed?"

Officer Brezhnev drew back. Taking a deep breath, he adjusted his bullet-proof vest and leaned over the Jag. The right hand back on the Glock. His eyes gathered strength, like two unsettled tornados about to touch down on a Missouri trailer park. He took a deep breath, and his voice settled into a civic and accommodating pedestrian tone.

"Well, Reeenardo… when I first read your license plate, I thought it read Herpes1, instead of Hermes1. Have an enjoyable day, and slow down before you catch something else," he said with an almost perceptible wink.

It was the first time he heard herpes used in public, in a one-liner forum while being the object of mockery. A drop in the ocean that would soon burst into a tsunami. The speeding ticket was the opening act of an Academy Award winning script. The movie, like this book, is a detailed description of how to prevent Genital Herpes from making a prisoner out of you, with an honorable mention on how to counteract its social stigma. Today I'm Herpes Free. My part in the script has ended; yours is about to start.

You're a Movie Star. The main character in your favorite film is faced with some great obstacle. The doctor has just informed him that the culture came back positive for Genital Herpes. What will you tell your fiancé? The wedding is next week. In all good motion pictures, something always goes wrong. If nothing goes wrong, there's no movie. The main character doesn't develop. The worst movies are pulled because they're uninspiring and don't develop. Lots of action, but no depth. That's why there's Facebook.

In inferior movies the problem or conflict is resolved on some external level. In *"Best Picture"* films, the main character faces some insurmountable obstacle. Faced with conflict, they grow, change, heal, and develop abilities they didn't have before. And then there are those memorable movies we can watch over-and-over again, because in them the main character also has an internal awakening, reconnecting them with their humanity and community. **"My Friend, the Enemy"** is like a movie script; how well you play the part is up to you.

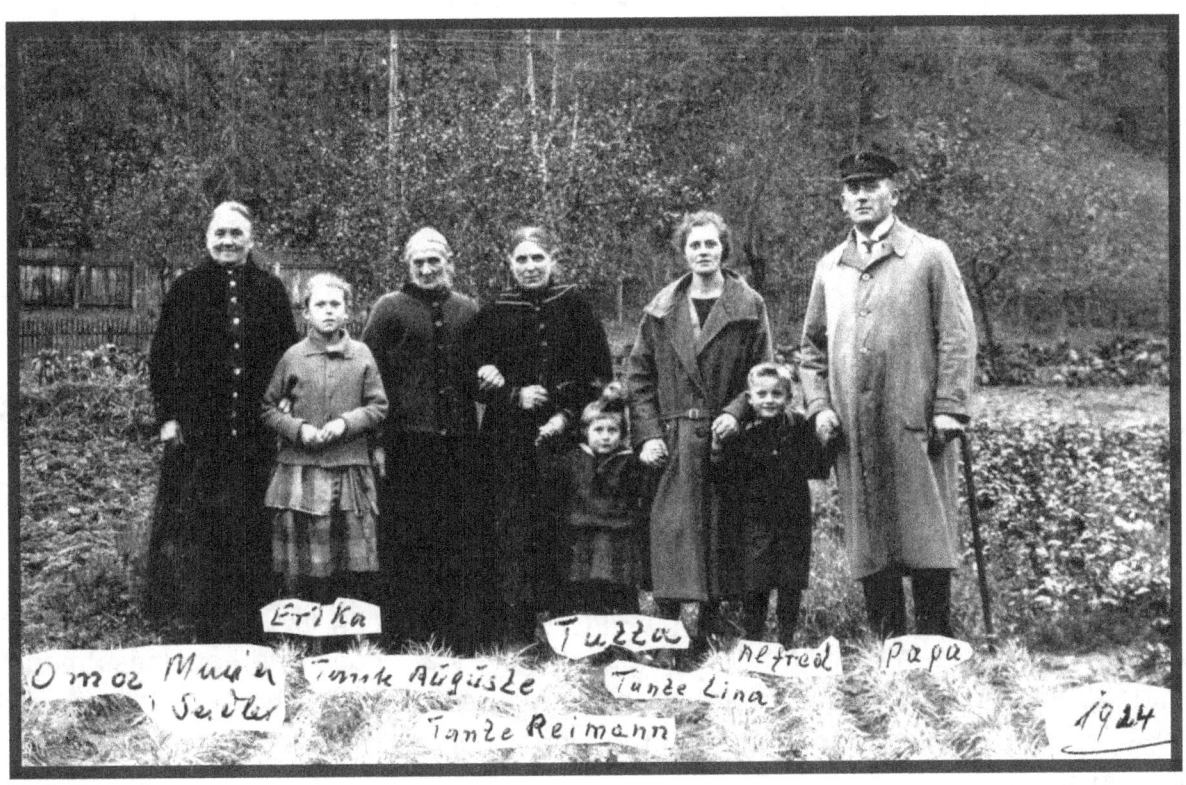

Family and Friends Survived the 1918 to 1920 Spanish Flu Pandemic

FOR YOUR INFORMATION: All <u>Underlined Hyperlinks</u> and their corresponding websites, offsite locations, and contacts are located at the end of this book under the heading: **Uniform Resource Locators URLs,** Websites: ***Genital Herpes, My Friend the Enemy.***

Introduction

"The universe is made of stories, not of atoms."
Muriel Rukeyser (1913 – 1980)

Few would argue that the current state of world affairs is a concern: Russia's attack of Ukraine; the infant formula shortage; rising fuel prices; COVID-19; and increased authoritarian censorship. That's why so many of us discount the small victories and tragedies of our ordinary lives. Through silence we often devalue our pain of how the herpes virus can diminish our capacity to live ordinary lives and open our hearts to love. Authoring this story is my way of telling the world, *"I was here, my life matters,"* and after you read this book you'll come to realize and believe so does yours.

From overcoming thoughts that your life will now be forever on hold, to leaving behind those moments and feelings of secluded sadness. Yes, you will learn to trust yourself again as you move into the recuperative process of enjoying life again. Realizing inner wisdom is far more important than information. And that peace and happiness means to suffer less. But neither is accessible until sorrow is transformed within. We are responsible for taking our Genital Herpes story and turning it right-side up. That's when our life will begin to change.

June 1981: HIV was first identified, and if not treated promptly can lead to AIDS (Acquired Immunodeficiency Syndrome). Currently there is no effective cure. Once people get HIV, they have it for life. But with proper medical care, it can be controlled.

July 2016: Zika is a virus transmitted by mosquitoes which typically causes a mild infection, fever, and rash.

May 2000: the Vladimir Putin *"virus"* was first unveiled. February 2022, the virus ordered Russian troops to invade Ukraine, *"in a major escalation of the Russo-Ukrainian conflict that began in 2014. The biggest assault on a European state since World War II. It caused the largest refugee crisis in Europe since World War II, with over 3.3 million Ukrainians* http://bit.ly/3zMwR2M *fleeing their country."*

February 16, 2022: the number of new COVID-19 cases worldwide dropped by nineteen percent (19%) percent in the past week, and despite being inexpensive, readily available, countless COVID treatments have been censored and suppressed in order to secure a global mass vaccination campaign. As of March 11, 2023, an estimated 270 million Americans had been vaccinated http://bit.ly/3MvOD1R and the Vaccine Adverse Event Reporting System (VAERS) data revealed seventy (70) deaths per day among vaccinated Americans. Some experts, including **Senator Ron Johnson** http://bit.ly/40V7asJ (R-Wis), who did not get vaccinated, think to have reliable VAERS statistics you would have to multiply this number dramatically to achieve real-world numbers. They believe the U.S. estimated daily death toll from COVID vaccines could be as high as 2,000 per day.

When hospitals were given large payments for COVID patients, every patient became a COVID-19 patient. At Elmhurst Hospital, New York, patients were labeled as COVID-19 even if they had a negative test and no symptoms. Most were placed on mechanical ventilation, which often killed them.

Physicians in Spain treated COVID patients with high doses of Vitamin D, and out of fifty (50) hospitalized COVID patients who were given oral vitamin D, only one needed treatment in the intensive care unit and there were no deaths. In comparison, among the 26-remaining COVID-19 patients who were not given vitamin D, 13 or 50% needed to be treated in the intensive care unit and two died. Unfortunately, at least 42% of the U.S. population is vitamin D deficient. Sixty percent (60%) of nursing home residents, and 76% of African Americans are deficient in this essential Vitamin. Why aren't we testing Covid-19 patients for vitamin D deficiency? And if patients are deficient, should they be treated with Vitamin D? Not treating them would be negligent, but then vitamin D is not a pharmaceutical drug.

What is a virus, and how does it infect us? Viral infections can occur almost anywhere in the body. Technically, a virus is an infectious agent that replicates inside a host, like plants, bacteria, and animals. That makes you, me, our friends, and pets fair game. Viruses constantly mutate into new variants. Some variants emerge and disappear, others like Genital Herpes persist.

U.S. COVID Cases: 01-21-20 to 03-12-23:

TOTAL CASES	THE LAST 7 DAYS	TOTAL DEATHS
103,191,231	120,118	1,126,060

https://covid.cdc.gov/covid-data-tracker/#cases_totalcases

or

https://tinyurl.com/2s4k9ys5

April 12, 2022: this book is not about Zika, HIV, or the COVID-19 virus, or an eBook with simple instructions, promises, then no more herpes outbreaks. No! In the past, all the so-called *"herpes-experts"* wanted to get right to the point with promises and easy-to-use systems that were simple and efficient. The problem? They never worked. Getting right to the point never stopped herpes or any virus from making its point.

Part of the healing process is *"patience"* instead of looking for the latest *"shortcut."* It's not out there, but the healing process is. Herpes, like COVID, is part of our living situation. Underneath the many conditions that make up our existence, there exists something deeper and more important. It's called *our life*. Who we truly are. The problem, we've covered it with so many labels, including herpes, we forget the importance of our *life*.

If we could refrain from labeling and mentally identifying with **Genital Herpes**, the virus for most people would be little more than a physical pain, irritation, discomfort, or minor disability. That's the part we acknowledge. Not the rest of the rubbish and baggage attached to it. Then instead of the *"Enemy"* using us, we use it to free ourselves from the bondage of discontent. Surrendering to our herpes situation in life does not transform its condition. Not directly. It transforms us. When we are transformed, our entire world changes, because the world is a reflection of the many labels and beliefs we attach to it.

The following paragraph may upset a few people. I know, because I get annoyed whenever I start to blame *"the situation,"* such as divorce, not enough money, or Genital Herpes. But then I realized they're not the problem. I'm the problem. Let me repeat and bring it closer to home. It's not herpes, or money, or divorce, we are the problem. Yes, that's hard to swallow but chew on it for a while. In time, you'll realize it's the only way out.

If you suffer from chronic herpes infections, or any kind of disability, do not feel that you have failed. Do not feel guilty or blame life for treating you unfairly. But do not blame yourself either. In fact, if anything bad happens in life, use *"the Enemy"* to gain a deeper understanding of who you are. Become an alchemist, transform herpes into healing, suffering into peace. Be your best *"Friend."* It's simple with the Hermes Protocol, but I've not said easy. If you're suffering from chronic Genital Herpes outbreaks and getting annoyed from what you've just read, it's a sign that herpes has maybe become part of your self-identity and you are now protecting yourself and the Enemy. The condition we label herpes has nothing to do with who we are. Whenever any kind of tragedy or misfortune strikes, please understand that there is another side to this hardship. We are only steps away from transforming the fertilizer of our life into a compost that will bear fruit, and the pain of fear into a jewel of peace.

For many who participate in a 12-Step Program, the first step is often called *"surrender."* That's not to say that you'll be happy in situations of surrender. You may not, but fear and pain can be transmuted into inner accord and serenity that is often called a *"Peace of God that passes all understanding."*

For most the predator is a mere physical annoyance. Sometimes worse, most of the time better. **But for some** outbreaks are more than a nuisance. They are a constant threat for emotional disturbances and the risk for more serious complications. What we all have in common is when our mind steps-in and amplifies a nuisance into a grievance.

Remedies for Genital Herpes:
1. Take suppressive anti-viral prescription medication.
2. Work with the mind.
3. Address the immune system and mind for physical and mental well-being.
4. Take a combination of natural protocols and supplements.

Your mission for the **Hermes Protocol (HP)** is to be open to change. Mine is to help you get in touch with your inner strength and to transform outbreaks into freedom. The difference with the **HP** is its two-pronged body-mind approach: to turn the enemy into a long-distance pen pal and replace frustration with serenity and health.

The Hermes Protocol is not a step-by-step, cookie-cutter, do-these-six-things, book. Or an example of the internet marketing mantra that less-sells-more. They have their place, but not today. Your life is not an eBook, neither is herpes. You ask, *"What time is it?"* The Hermes Protocol says, *"Forget the time, let's build a Genital Herpes time-bomb."* After suffering for thirty (30) years, today I'm six (6) years free.

The Hermes Protocol works by addressing:
1. A compromised immune system.
2. Necessary life-style changes.
3. Long-term emotional answers for peace of mind.
4. Natural protocols and supplements.

According to the World Health Organization, depression is now the leading cause of ill health and disability worldwide. http://bit.ly/2DDAKZ1Depression. Genital Herpes and depression is a relationship of dual causation and concern. *"Since sexually transmitted infections may trigger depression in susceptible persons, and psychological stress is associated with activation of Genital Herpes (HSV-2)."* In plain English, adults infected with HSV-2 are twice as likely to be depressed as adults who are not. http://bit.ly/2EgXbo2 Considering these bleak statistics, it would seem wise to be proactive about our mental and physical health, by looking at our lifestyle, immune system, diet, and supplements. That's what we'll do in the next 14 Chapters.

My Friend, the Enemy, details decades of experience, research, and testing many *"guaranteed"* herpes frauds, while maxing out *"credit-card-limits"* with ineffective supplements. In the process, I discovered the Hermes Protocol. There are going to be a few individuals who will fail with the Hermes Protocol. The truth is, I don't know why. That's the funny thing about healing. A person can do everything right and still fail. Even more bizarre, somebody can do everything wrong and still succeed. It's the law of alternative unpredictability. In Vegas it's called the *"odds."* The Weather Channel says there is a 90% chance. Orthodox medicine calls it idiopathic, or we're too idiotic to know why. Put them all together, it's life.

Many experts don't like talking about the unpredictability of results. How is it possible that the Hermes Protocol will work for most people and fail with some? Because healing and well-being often depend on commitment and mental attitude. Also, there's not much we can do to influence the unpredictability of destiny, except the following:

1. Be Prepared
2. Be Willing
3. Begin by Taking Action
4. Be Honest with Yourself

Good fortune, they say, favors the prepared.
Bad poverty, you say, prefers the unprepared. RH

Even though both political ideologies have promised and repeated themselves ad-nauseum to *"make America great again,"* in my lifetime I've NOT seen any resolve in abandoning military conflict, solving poverty, or improving the human condition. If anything is going to change, it's going to be up to us. Just as we've come to appreciate the importance that sex must be good for both partners, we need to recognize we're all harmed by our indifference, whether it's Genital Herpes or general hunger.

Please, let me know if you find any mistakes, *errors-of-omission*, or ignored essential information. Email **RHermes1@gmail.com** and I will make appropriate changes at the next revision. The only tolerance I would ask. Please forgive my long-windedness and redundant nature. English is my second language, and sometimes German's rambling language structure interferes.

Chronic Genital Herpes infections are also not a Valtrex deficiency. If you're looking for a silver bullet to eliminate herpes outbreaks, take the nuclear option—suppressive antiviral therapy—and be done with it. Then there is no reason to read further. The **Hermes Protocol (HP)** is about improving immune function, healing emotions, and supporting the mind. A much healthier, less toxic, and more enduring approach to alleviate outbreaks.

A few thoughts before we begin. I hope you'll forgive me for mostly using the male pronoun to stand for both genders. Saying he or she over-and-over again is a distraction. Also, please try to resist fear when herpes pays you a visit. Turn away from any mental chatter that says you *'lack.'* Run away from the inner voice that tells you that you *'fall-short.'* And shut down the *'they win, I lose'* herpes mental program. Resist your 'outbreak-brains' constant negative chatter by sifting it through a filter of realism. Live less seriously. Not by ignoring the facts-of-life, but by putting the past behind you. Like Shakespeare said, *"I would rather have a fool make me merry, than experience make me sad."* Peace of mind is a day-to-day effort.

PART ONE: IN THE BEGINNING

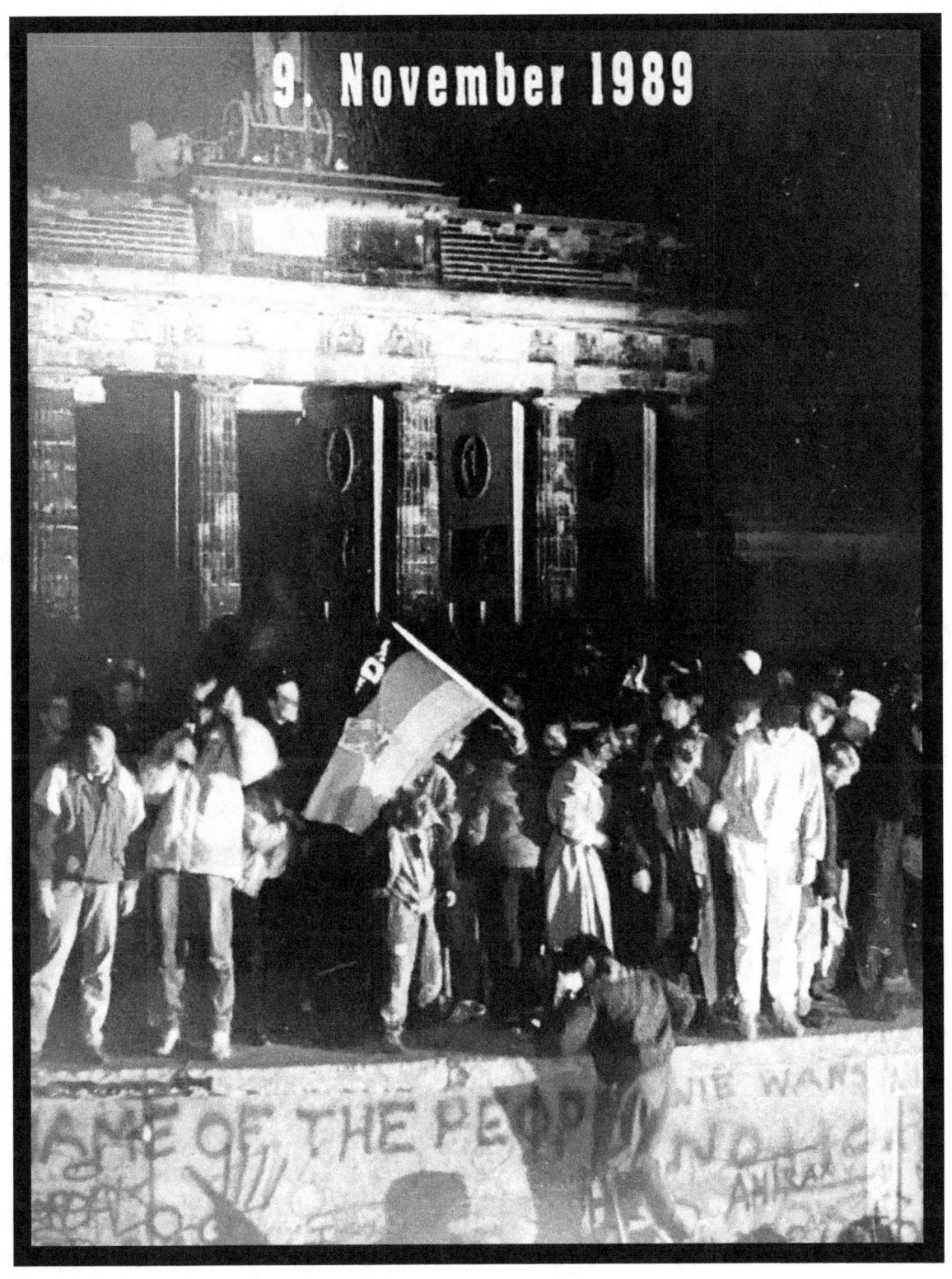

Chapter 1: Rx for Humor

"When life give you lemons, just be glands it wasn't Genital Herpes." – R. Hermes

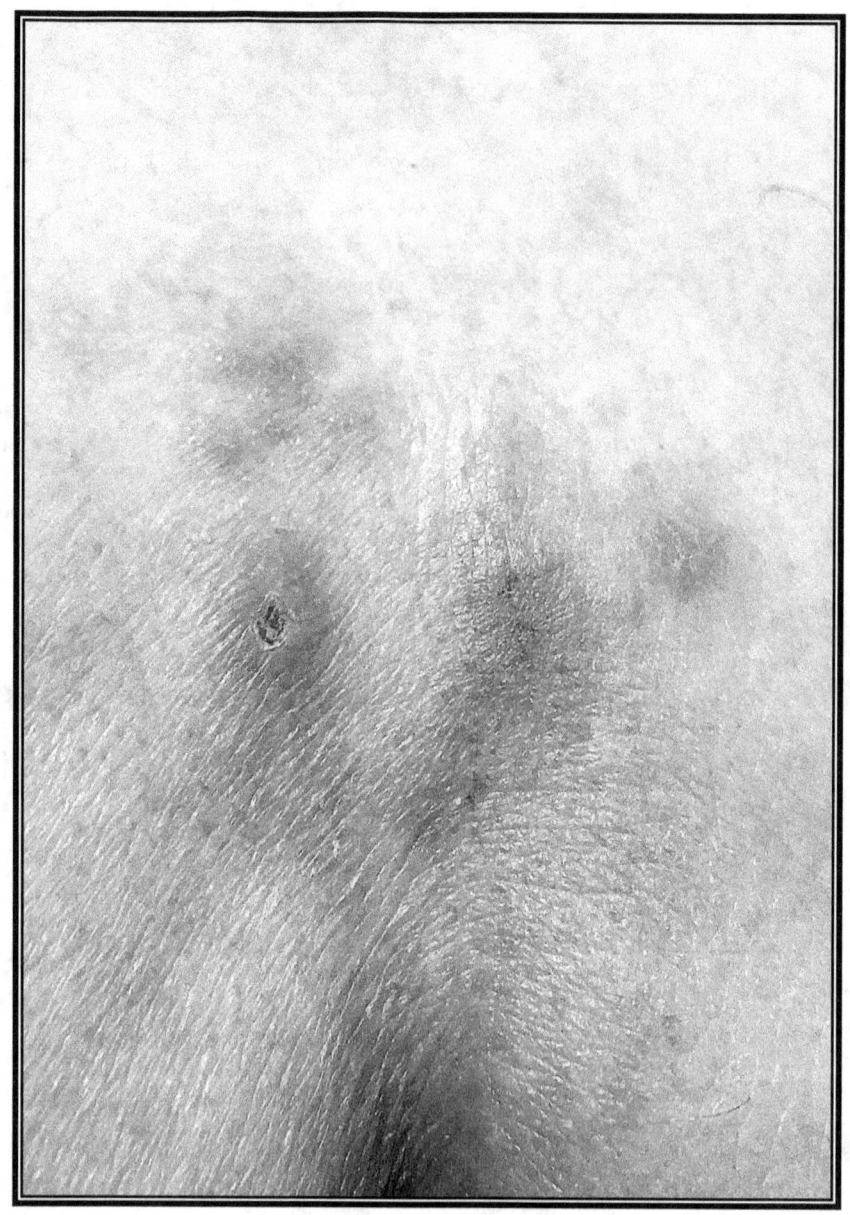

2016 Sacral Herpes

A. Herpes1 vs. Hermes1

A couple of Genital Herpes infections a year were no big deal. However, in time their frequency and severity increased. It reached hurricane crescendo in 2016 with seventy-plus (70+) outbreaks, including a serious complication which even alarmed my stoic doctors. Sometimes herpes is more than a blistery inconvenience. **Eczema Herpeticum** is a serious infection where the viral hunter enlists eczema to do its mischief. A full-blown hurricane, with its distorted pain, sacral discomfort, and turbulent nights, it paled compared to the anxiety it created when I *"Googled"* Eczema Herpeticum.

It was the '80s when the Greek god Apollo went on a warpath in Orange County, California. Taking aim, he shot a quiver of *"Herpesviridae"* at my lips and privates. It became their playground for the next 40 years, while they became my nemesis.

It's been challenging at times. Genital Herpes was part of the reason my wife and I divorced. No different than other couples who are in pain and suffering with their own demons from more serious diseases. If what I've gone through will resonate and help someone put Genital Herpes in remission, and a smile back on their face, then my experience, time, and effort in authoring this book was time well spent and a blessing of great proportion. Heartfelt appreciation to all the internet surfers, bloggers, and authors, whose stories are the fabric, binding, and support that bind this book.

B. Berlin L.A. Express

As you might have guessed, with a first name like Reinhard, I'm not a good *ol'* boy but a *guten ol'* Kraut from Germany. Born in Berlin, Germany, after World War II, living conditions were similar to the Hobbit's carpet-bombed-out Mordor. Food was scarce, blood-sausage a treat, medical facilities *"Absent With Out Leave,"* and undetonated bombs our parent's nightmare. If postwar stress was the catalyst for Dad divorcing Mom, a more persuasive reason Mom was a wee bit alcoholic, like the Titanic a bit unlucky.

Escape: in 1956 we found our way out of Berlin's rubble. Mom, Oma, and I packed our suitcases and immigrated to the good old USA. My Aunt Krista had led the way when she married GI Joe, who she met working at the U.S. Army Post Exchange. When GI Joe rotated stateside to California, Aunt Krista sent for us ASAP.

Eight years later, July 1964, before my eighteenth birthday, I dropped out of high school, and joined the U.S. Army. During basic training at Fort Ord, California, a Spinal Meningitis epidemic swept through our base, crippling, or killing hundreds of trainees. I was fortunate. Hospitalized six (6) weeks, two in an iron lung, I survived with double pneumonia. My roommate, Carney, and many others were not so fortunate. Many died within days after onset of symptoms. Unable to stop the Meningitis epidemic, they closed Fort Ord in 1965.

C. 80's Wannabees

In the 1980s most Orange County (OC) hippie-wannabes didn't know or care about the difference between Genital Herpes and gentle hippies from the San Francisco Bay Area. Doing the OC bar scene, many of us confused the flowering of *"free-love"* for *"free-sex."* Then heaved a sigh of reprieve that the diagnosis was just a plain old STD or HSV, and not HIV/AIDS.

Medicine's use of *acronyms* for Socially Transmitted Diseases (STDs), like HSV, HIV and AIDS, seems to make them less infectious, more benign, and sterile, than their reality. Then something unexpected happened that put a damper on the OC nightlife. In 1982, *Time Magazine* ran the *Scarlett Letter H* cover story, and the *LA Times* reported on the deadly AIDS epidemic. But the *"nail"* in OC's nightlife was a 1986 Orange Coast Magazine article that reported, *"165 cases of AIDS… of which 87 died."* http://bit.ly/2rKxVUA

The OC curtain fell hard on the "beautiful people." When we heard a friend or acquaintance symptomatic with any kind of rash or "itch," we were quick to gossip, blame, and bestow the finger on our "free-love" brothers in the Bay Area, who we blamed for our night-life-crisis. Most of us were at the pre-grunting stage of consciousness. Our emotional dashboards frequently flashed empty when it came to *"humility or compassion,"* but always seemed to have a full tank of *"judgement, criticisms, or condemnation."* The venom dissipated once we heard the test results, heaving a big sigh of relief it was only HSV and not HIV.

In our enclave of pretentious *'booshwazees'* wannabes, play-act-dealers, and never-graduate from college students, most of us were only after-hour hippie make-believes, too entrenched in the O.C. Disco-Culture to ever leave home without our AMEX. Although a few smoked or snorted like hippies, the majority just drank and drove like plain ol' garden variety DUIs. It was on one of those nights. No more and no less pretentious or repetitious than many before, that I said good night to my friend Chris and closed the door to another forgettable chapter of my life.

According to Stanford University, herpes has been breaking down doors since ancient Greece. But its persistent predatory stigma didn't get traction until the hippie movement and its sexual association with HIV/AIDS. http://stanford.io/2FoKxT5

The '80s were challenging times, not only for main street, but also medical boulevard. From yuppie homemakers to infectious disease specialists, everyone seemed as perplexed about herpes as they were about AIDS, with more fear and uncertainty than knowledge. Everyone that was anyone suddenly wanted to be tested *"to be sure."* If a medical assistant suspected you were positive, they put on a hermetically sealed space suit and gave you the sign of the cross. More accurate news broadcasts were heard from the stalls of public restrooms than the halls of medicine. In retrospect, much of the stigma and fear was orchestrated by those who benefited the most. And the sales of antiviral medications have never slowed. Neither has their pricing. I wonder? Today, we have COVID-19. Not much has changed.

Project Aspect still blames the herpes' stigma on big pharma's hyped antiviral drug marketing campaign of the '70s and early '80s. But unlike COVID-19 today or HIV yesterday, Genital Herpes is still the *"largest epidemic no one wants to talk about,"* wrote Eric Sabo of the *New York Times,* and *LA Times* headline declared Genital Herpes a *"Sexual Sore Spot That's Spreading"* and *"roaring through parts of Orange County like an unwanted dinner guest."*

D. Stigma & Disclosure

Increased stigma and psychosocial burden associated with Genital Herpes in the early 1980s prompted the creation of support groups, dating services, and social networks that are still strong today. The American Social Health Association (ASHA) established a Herpes Resource Center (HRC) and a large network of support groups. ASHA serves many roles: *information, support for those with herpes, and a public voice*. Herpes has a unique stigma among Sexually Transmitted Diseases (STDS). Few poke fun at people with HIV/AIDS because it's perceived as a serious disorder. Chlamydia, syphilis, crabs, scabies, and gonorrhea are now and then the target of shaggy-dog jokes, but these STDS have for the most part been cured (until recently). And people don't endure them for long.

Genital Herpes on the other hand, is thought to be incurable. A disease of the immoral and cheating types. Therefore, they deserve it, making it a popular gag topic. Regardless of where the stigma came from, pig pharma, stand-up comedy, late night TV, films, or the Fake-News-Media. They all keep it alive. After being diagnosed, Genital Herpes sufferers fall somewhere between *"my life is over"* or *"it makes sense."* A few, like me, detach and become conspiracy applicants. Denial and anger were at the top of my emotional response.

It can be confusing wondering, and thinking back about who might have infected you, and in turn, who did you infect? I don't know about today, but at the beginning of the *"free-sex"* era it wasn't important to keep track of who you slept with. STDS were not that complicated or much of an issue. But that's changed. Today with COVID-19 it's more challenging than ever. Genital Herpes is not the issue it used to be because COVID has made intimate contact difficult. Instead of condoms we wear masks and keep six feet apart. I know some men profess to be well endowed but not large or long enough to disobey social distancing.

Throw in a batch of fear and guilt, thinking that you may give the gift *"that-keeps-on-giving"* to someone else, and a whole treasure trove of mental and emotional issues are composting waiting to surface and make a stink. One of the most difficult concerns is whether to dialogue with people from your past, wondering if they'd already passed it on to the next generation. That's why disclosure issues are a frequent discussion topic on herpes dating sites. In retrospect, being on the side of truthfulness and concern over others, resonates and aligns with truth and *"divine wisdom."* Also, personal transformation starts with honesty, including Genital Herpes.

Whether to disclose too soon or too late? Or wait for that textbook moment when they see you as a person, not a creep or victim. Good luck with that! Thank goodness that Scarlett H people have few issues when it comes to disclosing to family and friends. Most are supportive and sympathetic. The most feared disclosure struggles involve romantic situations, which some avoid altogether. *"All this insecurity, discouragement, rejection, tears, anger, counseling, suicidal tendencies, humiliation, shame, and isolation is caused by the stigma of a skin condition that for most people doesn't show up at all or only a couple of times a year."*—The Atlantic

The stigma of Genital Herpes created by our mind, may not survive the facts. But why confuse delusion and tweets with facts? *Humpty Trumpty and Hilariously* seldom did. So why should we? Try to keep in mind that herpes, although it can consume us, is only a small part of who and what we are. It also helps **not** *to label every situation or event* that occurs in our lives as either good or bad.

This is tough to overcome, or even to acknowledge, because so much of our everyday life is spent that way. From the *"rainy"* weather, the *"slow"* line at Starbucks, or the *"cold"* temperature in our office. Herpes is not good or bad. Herpes just is. Yes, I have herpes. Yes, it's unfortunate. But it's also undesirable to have spinal stenosis, a compromised immune system, nail fungus, a detached wife, and a variable mortgage. And by the way, the temperature in the office is… blah, blah, blah. On and on and on it goes, where it will end everybody knows. No one gets to be happy. Unless of course you *"ask-your-doctor,"* and take a pharmaceutical drug.

In summary: try not to turn every herpes outbreak into a dramatic mental script in which you play the victim, herpes the villain, while looking to be rescued. Don't divide your herpes outbreak life into rewards or threats, friends or foes, and outcome as loss or gain. Unhappiness is seldom a result of a single situation or events like herpes outbreaks, but many small errors in judgment repeated every day for many years. Do not panic or succumb to the blows of outbreaks or delegate your accountability to your partner or doctor. Practice 'practical-optimism,' not by pretending or ignoring that herpes exists, but by living in the moment and putting the past behind you. Don't waste energy on carrying grudges or judging. Resentments and revenge are the most unproductive way of spending the present moment and could lead to even more outbreaks.

E. Double Edged Support

Genital Herpes support groups are double-edged guillotines. Yes, they may help you to move beyond herpes, and *"made us feel less unique. It puts things into perspective. It helped make me feel that I'm not a virus; I'm Reinhard."* However, they can also reinforce and contribute to the herpes stigma by creating a virus group identity, further ostracizing us from society and humanity. They can help people cope and adjust, but only to the point where it integrates them back into the flow of life, not away from it. Herpes contributes to that enough. We don't need to create more separation by excluding the infected person, as if he's the disease, not herpes. Do not compound isolation by denying that we are part of a complicated and often frustrating social order. Herpes only plays a small part, though it often wants and demands all our full attention.

Herpes for extra credit. Life is a classroom. A required course, not an elective. I don't have a choice whether to take it or not, or even when to take it. Every morning when I wake up, school is in session. It doesn't matter whether I pull the covers back over my head, class is still in session. With or without me. There is no inclement weather or sick days. Life is not based on a grading system, even though the media and powers-to-be want us to buy into that story line. Life gives a *"pass"* just for showing up, or *"no-pass"* and *"do-over"* if we decide to be a no-show. There is no failing, but on occasion it feels like fumbling. The Genital Herpes curriculum was a constant do-over. The lessons are long and painful. I often stayed after school until I learned enough to be Herpes Free.

The only other way out is by not opting out, but learning everything we can about our herpes' triggers. Like you're doing now by reading this book. Many of us have an authority problem. We don't like being told to show up. Let alone what to do or how to do it. But if we want to master any subject, or learn to play an instrument, it's easier with a *"guidebook"* and lessons. Congratulations! You now have a manual for Genital Herpes. Let it guide you. The curriculum will be easier and less stressful. Then all that's left is to get up every morning and practice, practice, practice. Until one day you sit down at the piano and stop playing *"chopsticks"* but start composing your own music and realize you're not squirming in your seat. The itching has stopped.

Herpes is a part of your curriculum; otherwise, there would be no need to read this workbook. For others, their syllabus might be obesity, bankruptcy, cancer, divorce. What a laboratory? I want to thank those who have been instrumental in combating herpes and never giving up. Without their exploration, persistence, and guiding wisdom, I would still be of the *"Why me?"* mindset. It's not been easy. At times difficult, but I've led a productive and blessed life, filled with all its *"normal"* trials and misfortunes, including getting divorced.

I'd like to forget a few embarrassing moments, when my social interactions were distorted and awkward because they were filtered through a herpes looking glass. But, as the French Huguenots would say, *"Sheet happens!"* You've got that right. I've had it *'happens'* there, too. *Ouch!* I've learned a few things that will benefit you physically and emotionally. Authoring a book about herpes is not as painful as having weekly flare-ups. There's not much to writing. I sit in front of the computer, cut open my right wrist vein, and let the words bleed into colorful pages of flora.

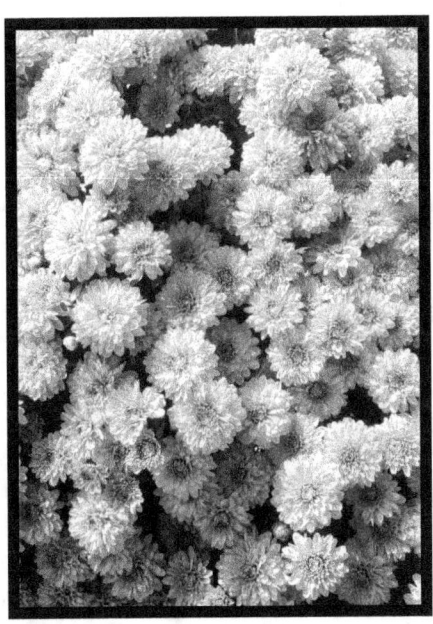

F. Pregnancy

1983: two years after getting married, Jennifer was pregnant with our second child. Toward the end of her pregnancy, she suffered several Genital Herpes outbreaks. The stress of pregnancy exasperated her vaginal rashes. Even in the eighties ('80s) the medical community was conscious of how serious *"neonatal herpes'* could be for the baby if the mother had the herpes virus in her birth canal during delivery. Although it was a rare occurrence (one per 3,000 to 20,000 live births), Jenny and I were anxious.

Newly infected mothers do not have time to build antibodies. There is also little in the way of protection for the infant, making him or her at a much higher risk for a serious infection. Even though taking Acyclovir during the last month of pregnancy was an option, and presumably safe, we hesitated for fear of exposing our baby to its side effects. If pregnant and infected with Genital Herpes, make sure to tell your doctors. Active infections can lead to miscarriages or premature delivery. You'll be offered antivirals toward the end of your pregnancy. They can reduce the risk of symptoms and transmitting the disease to the baby. If stressed, and still unsure at delivery, consider a 'C-section.' Please follow the link. *"I'm pregnant.* http://bit.ly/2nhZrUACDC *How could Genital Herpes affect my baby?"*

Jennifer decided on a Cesarean. October 26, 1983, we were both overjoyed with the birth of our cheerful and healthy boy, *'artistic'* Elliot. The doctors were conscientious and examined Jenny before and after delivery for any signs of herpes symptoms. They did the same for "delicate-Elliot." Thirty-four years later, on January 22, 2018, my son, Elliot and his wife, Marissa gave birth to Nolan Hermes at 11:11 AM. The mystery and profound joy in the *"Circle-of-Life"* as it unfolds.

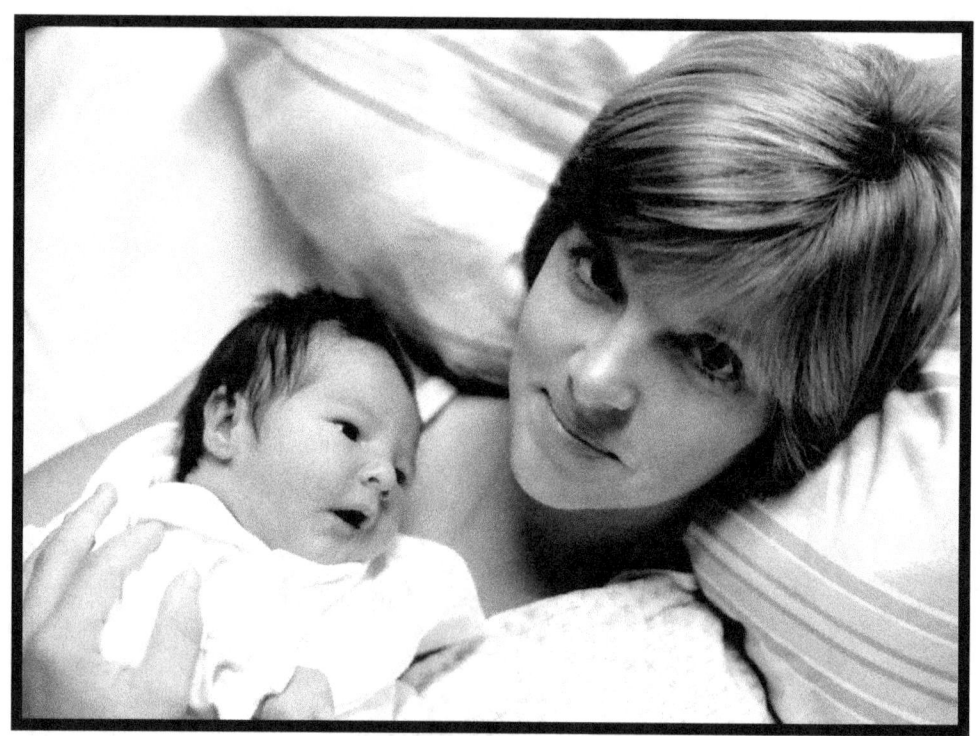

Jenny's Delight in Motherhood with her Joy, Elliot.

G. Know Your Cause

Immune deficiency health issues can often be found in overdosing on a *"free"* lifestyle, endless rounds of antibiotics, or dozens of suppressive symptom medications. Throughout the never-ending testing process, my doctors kept repeating their "idiopathic" mantra. *"We're not sure, but let's run this other test. Meanwhile, take this (drug); it might help with (name the symptom)."* My primary doctors never did find out or *"know the cause."*

But in May 2011, while undergoing a nerve conduction study, the Neurologist thought out-loud that I might be suffering from *"Primary Immunodeficiency,"* in view of recent infections and heart issues. His suspicions were confirmed six (6) months later with lab tests. I'm immune compromised. They don't know why but most likely from serving in the U.S. Army around nuclear munitions without proper protective gear.

IV IG don't know: the Neurologist's recommendation was IVIG infusion therapy. Because of its cost and uncertainty, I looked for an alternative treatment. In March 2012, I discovered **Low Dose Naltrexone**, most often known by its acronym, **LDN**. A three mg (3-mg) prescription calmed my immune system, reduced heart palpitations, and decreased herpes outbreaks from every 2 or 3 weeks to every few months.

Intravenous Immunoglobulin (IVIG): is used to treat various autoimmune diseases, infectious, neuropathic, and idiopathic illnesses. The body's immune system normally makes enough antibodies to fight germs that cause infections, but with immune deficiency, the body can't make enough. They seldom know the cause but are glad to treat its symptoms. The problem with symptomatology, it's most often idiopathic, a disease or condition that arises spontaneously for which the cause is unknown. In plain language, scientists and doctors don't know. So, they guess. The out-of-pocket *"guesstimate"* for the idiopathic treatment? A four-dose course of IVIG for a 155-lb. person was about $25,000 per month. The problem, I weighed 190, but it wouldn't have mattered if I weighed 45 pounds. Out-of-pocket expenses were estimated to be $10,000 to $15,000 a month. That's if the insurance company approved it, and then, *"We're not even sure it'll work, but let's try it for at least 3 months."*

A study at Harvard University http://bit.ly/2rIviTlHarvard indicated that medical expenses represent 62% of all personal bankruptcies. The study set aside the myth that most bankrupt individuals didn't have health insurance, when in fact, 78% did. It finally put to rest the fairytale that medical bills only affect the uninsured.

It takes guts: our gut mucosa connects with the largest population of immune cells in the body. Known as gastrointestinal immune cells, which originate in the lymphoid branch of the immune system. Their aim is to attack harmful invaders. Guess what *"anti-life-biotics"* do to your gut bacteria? The take-home mantra: if you want a healthy immune system, *"take care of your pocketbook, so you can take care of your gut."* It's hard to say how many antibiotic prescriptions I've taken over the course of my lifetime. Best guess is less than one hundred, but more than fifty. The most damaging and difficult treatments were for TB (tuberculosis) in 2002 and Triple-H-Pylori therapy. I didn't finish the TB protocol, because of too many adverse side effects.

The *powers-to-be* weren't even sure I had TB. There were no symptoms, only a positive TB skin test. Everybody freaked. Later, I found out this response is most often a false-positive response to being vaccinated! But when in doubt, prescribe the most virulent *"anti-life-biotics"* possible. They say *"Scheisse-Happens,"* except when it doesn't. And that's what didn't happen to me after the TB protocol and second H-Pylori therapy. I got plugged up, BIG TIME, and the problem didn't budge for many years, and years, and years, just like **My Friend, the Enemy.**

H. Grim Side Effects

The following is a short-list of pharmaceuticals that were prescribed over a three-year (3-year) period. I didn't include most *antibiotics* because there were too many. At the time, no one thought there was a need for concern, including my doctors. Today we know better. Every time I walked into a dentist's office, along with a lollipop, I got a dose of antibiotics. Mitral Valve Prolapse, an irregular heartbeat, palpitations, and/or shortness of breath required dental antibiotics before anyone said, *"Open-up."*

3-years of Rx for Better Health:

1. **Acyclovir** 400 MG: 3X a Day AS NEEDED
2. **Nystatin** & Fluconazole 500,000: 3 Times a day, Candida
3. **Antifungal** Ketonazole Cream 2%
4. **Clotrimazole:** 10 MG Troche for mouth
5. **LDN Cream:** At night before bedtime, Herpes-Immune
6. **Liothyronine:** 5 MCG taken 1/2 Tablet Twice Daily
7. **Levothyroxine:** 50 MCG every AM
8. **Armour Thyroid:** 90 MG
9. **Testosterone Gel:** 1 Packet AM
10. **Minocycline:** 100 MG 3X a week, M-W-F
11. **Fluconazole:** 200 MG 1X a Day
12. **Acarbose:** 25 MG 3X a Day Start of Each Meal
13. **Baclofen:** 10 MG 6X a Day AS NEEDED
14. **Cortisone/Nys Cream:** 2X a Day
15. **Gabapentin:** 300 MG 3X a Day
16. **Etodolac:** 400 MG 2X a Day
17. **Cyclobenzaprine:** 10 MG 3X a Day
18. **Prednisone:** 10 MG 4X a Day
19. **Hyomax-SL:** 125 MG AS NEEDED
20. **Buspirone HCL:** 5 MG 2 to 3X a Day
21. **AndroGel:** 1 Packet Daily to Skin

Grim Statistics about Rx Risks:

1. **16% of hospital admissions** related to adverse Rx reactions.
2. **Fourth leading cause of death** in the U.S. is prescription drugs.
3. **70 potential adverse reactions** in the average American drug.
4. **106,000 deaths per year** from Rx drugs properly prescribed.
5. **Only 10,000 deaths per year** from illegal drugs.

October 2009: after several rounds of antibiotics for a severe tooth infection, my future-wife and I were looking for a new place to live. We found a secluded and attractive townhome in Mission Viejo, CA. While going through our walk-through, we decided to test drive the carpets skid-mark durability, crossing the finish line in a walk-in bedroom closet. That's the last thing I remember before bumping into the main entrance at Mission Viejo Hospital. According to my wife, I *"behaved"* no less normal than usual. Including being able to drive on the freeway under 80 MPH. But afterwards, she said I kept repeating myself, repeating myself with, *"Where were we just now? Where were we just now?"*

It's when I got confused using the condominium gate-opener that she got concerned. In the Emergency Room at Mission Viejo Hospital, they diagnosed me with **Transient Global Amnesia (TGA).** During episodes of TGA, you're NOT able to recall recent events. Moments of *here-and-now* go *"poof"* into *there-and-gone* into who knows where. Like the marriage vows we took, *"…from this day forward, …. blah, blah, blah, blah… for poorer, in sickness and in health, until death do us part."* Gone.

Getting married is stressful. Many couples resort to a preventative dose of anti-stress-biotics, which might explain the mini-Transient Global Amnesia (TGA) epidemic sweeping our nation as couples experience *"marriage-vow"* TGA. When their marriage falls apart, they keep repeating the same questions over-and-over again. *What just happened to us?* They can't remember, or their vows.

I was kept overnight. The next day the ER doc told me that I was fortunate it was **TGA** and not a **TIA** stroke. He smiled and wished me, *"Good Luck."* A few days later I had another minor event. Fortunately, Transient Global Amnesia is rare, mostly harmless, and unlikely to happen again, or happen again. My episodes were short-lived, and afterward my memory was okay. I've had no re-occurrence, but I can't say that about *"My Friend, the Enemy."* He was a constant reminder of the TGA incident whenever I repeated myself with *"Oh, no, not again. Oh, no, not again."*

Hermes Protocol helps restore health, reduces, or eliminates herpes outbreaks, and allows a person to live in peace in an insane world, with or without taking vows. But the best part for those close to me. I've stopped repeating myself.

I. The ol' Mule

When I finished the **Hermes Protocol,** my Genital Herpes infections dropped from over 40+ in 2016, to four in 2017, and none in 2018. As in *zero* or *not one*. If outbreaks have made you a prisoner inside your own body and you feel confused, humiliated, and want to hurt that special someone. Welcome to the world of *"specialness,"* and *"It's not fair."*

Here's what a wise university graduate professor once told me when I had one of my *"it's-so-unfair"* tantrums. She said, *"Whoever told you that life is fair?"* It was an **"Ah-Ha"** defining moment. At the time I didn't think her advice was very sympathetic or helpful, in view of the self-imposed pain I'd put myself through. So, I did what every good American does when they feel pain. I self-medicated with a *"brownie."* It was the '70s. Today, that advice still rings clear and is my go-to bedrock memory whenever I think life is "unfair." I started healing on many levels when I traded my fist waving *"why-me?"* outbreak battle-cry for one of acceptance and "why not me?" And I'd also remember *"The Farmer and the ol' Mule"* parable.

The Farmer and the ol' Mule

Once upon a time there was a farmer who had an ol' mule that fell into a dry well. The farmer sympathized with the ol' mule but decided the mule and the well were not worth saving. So, he called his neighbors and they decided to bury the ol' mule in the well. Killing two problems in one. Well, so he thought. The farmer and his friends shoveled dirt, shovel-full after shovel-full, into the well, and onto the mule. But every time a shovel of dirt landed on the ol' mule, he just kept shaking-it-off and stepping up.

No matter how painful the shovel loads, or frustrating the situation seemed, the ol' mule just kept shaking off the dirt and stepping up. *Shaking it off and stepping up.* Worn out and pummeled with dirt, the ol' mule finally stepped up and out of the well into green pastures. *"Oh well,"* thought the farmer, as he watched his ol' mule grazing in the meadow. The mule slowly turned toward the farmer, and to his amazement, the farmer thought he saw the ol' mule smile. Like the mule, life's classroom often throws dirt on us. Then do like the ol' mule. Shake it off and step on up, until you can walk into greener pastures. If you're one of the unlucky ones, and outbreaks have shoveled insecurities, depression, shame, and guilt into your well of self-worth, remember the ol' mule and keep shaking it off and stepping up, until you can transcend into greener pastures.

Internal Emotional Struggles: often manifest themselves externally as disease. Undue stress can trigger Genital Herpes outbreaks, and the infection often perpetuates the cycle by causing more stress, creating a painful boomerang affect. Lifting the veil of secrecy can be effective for many Genital Herpes sufferers. Sharing the diagnosis or educating others, especially during the current COVID-19 time, are important steps to integrating Genital Herpes back into society and eliminating its stigma. Yes, I have herpes, but I'm not alone. Today is a new day, a new beginning. Although this is my personal story, it's a collective accounting. Yours, mine and the many whose history contributed to formulating the Hermes Protocol. Today I live in détente with *"My Friend, the Enemy."* The curriculum of *"shake it off and step-on-up."*

Chapter 2: Living Sick, Dying Young

"Divine wisdom does not judge, criticize, or condemn. It gets even." – RH

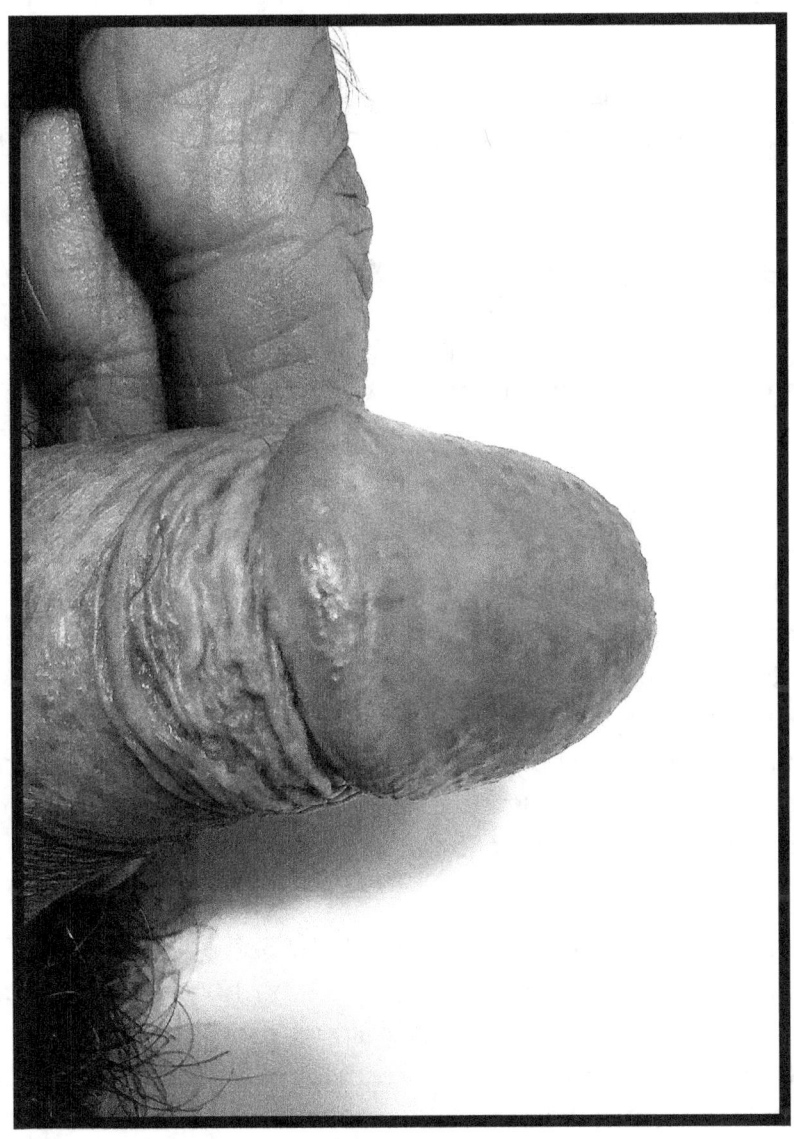

Genital Herpes

A. Negativity Bias

One of the first things to realize about your Genital Herpes experience and trauma is *"You survived."* Acknowledging *"I survived"* can be a news flash to the psyche and nervous system. That's not to imply that we try to convince ourselves that Genital Herpes is a blessing or a gift, but to think of outbreaks as "givens." It makes it easier not to rationalize or blame outbreak frustrations on anyone else. If something is a *given*, it just is. Don't deny or pretend herpes doesn't exist. Start by acknowledging it, then have the best life possible going forward.

That's not easy in an age of blame and shame, contrived effects, and social isolation. The concept of healing our pain and treating ourselves with compassion has gotten a bad rap. Conformist moral thinking goes something like this. *"Loving ourselves is narcissistic, selfish, self-indulgent, and the supreme fantasy of a disguised ego looking out for number one."* I don't speak French, but I know a few German words, and my answer to that ridiculous notion is, *"Bullshit!"* Ooops, that's not German, that's Houston. In fact, if we have a chronic disease, like herpes, the opposite is true. If the airplane cabin pressure dropped on the way to San Jose, no one would call us selfish if we secured our oxygen mask first before helping another.

No matter what the disease or outer circumstance, to honor oneself is to come into harmony with life itself, including our family, friends, and everyone else. I'll discuss that process in more detail later in the chapter: *"Out of Love."* For most of us, the experiences we have are a mixed bag of both positive and negative events. But scientists who study human behavior tell us that we have a *'negativity-bias.'* It makes us especially alert to danger and threat. That way we don't become lunchmeat for a crouching saber-tooth tigress. A doormat for a mob of virulent *"Black Friday"* shoppers, or flypaper to marauding bacteria and replicating viruses. Because of this negativity-bias, we can feel lost or discouraged from chronic herpes infections. Not being able to evoke positive memories, feelings of joy, and comfort.

Yes, herpes at times can be serious and debilitating. But while we're suffering, and going through the healing process, don't forget to live. Being herpes *"free"* is a process, not a switch. Don't put life on hold because of the pain or keep mourning the loss of your Life Before Herpes (LBH). The consequences are more detrimental than outbreaks. Life on hold is a *"choke-hold"* for those who live with a relentless negative-biased partner. It's OK to feel OK, even if we experience one outbreak after another. We don't have to hurt every moment of every day. Take those times to smile whenever they happen. It will get better.

I used to make a *"big-deal"* about almost everything. *"Doing-human,"* I exaggerated most of my problems. Genital Herpes was no exception. A saner approach to life is to have an attitude of honoring things, but not making them *so important.* Maintaining a feeling of *glad to be alive* yet acknowledging herpes outbreaks with an open mind. That doesn't mean we sit back and do nothing. We stay proactive about taking the necessary steps to be **"Herpes-Free."** We don't belittle or make light of our problems but neither fan them into an inferno of *"big-deals."*

B. Chronic Outbreaks

The Hermes Protocol (HP) addresses the immune system, nutrition, diet, supplementation, lifestyle, mindfulness, and detoxification. Given the right conditions, the body will restore itself to a state of dynamic equilibrium called *"good-health."*

Three Adversaries of Good Health:
1. **Deficiency**
2. **Toxicity**
3. **Uncontrolled Mind**

From minor outbreaks to Herpeticum, the Hermes Protocol (HP) set me *"Free."* My prison-break-strategy worked. I've been on outbreak parole since May 2017, as opposed to 2016, when I was locked-up in solitary herpetic confinement for over 40 weeks. Maybe the HP can transform your negativity bias and grant you an early parole and freedom? I've been fortunate; even in the depth of quarantine, I kept faith. It's not been a party. But it made living with my herpes cell mate less burdensome and the protocols easier. Ninety percent (90%) of the Hermes Protocol is *"physical"* therapies, supplements, and procedures. The superglue that holds them all together is the mind. The least expensive, most powerful, misunderstood healing remedy in the HP. Period.

This book serves those who are distressed. Whose outbreaks have cornered them into a cell of frustration and feelings of futility. If the sexual predator has made you a prisoner of a truncated life, the HP can grant your pardon. But there is a price for freedom: to be more hands-on and make lifestyle changes that can prove difficult.

As far as mental and spiritual matters are concerned, I'm not asking you to judge or believe them. You just need to use them. In fact, you don't even have to welcome them, and some you may resist. None of that matters or decreases their effectiveness. Whatever your reactions may be, use them. They will not interfere with any of your beliefs or values.

IMPORTANT: many people keep looking and hoping to find a *"by-the-numbers"* cure. Do these six steps and *"no-more-herpes."* There is a simpler way. Remember my suggestion? It's simple. Take suppressive Rx antiviral therapy. If it works, great! It didn't work for me and caused unpleasant side effects.

Herpes-Freedom is independence from a lifestyle that compromises the immune system. With all its mental formations of anger, misery, and delusion. It's past time to unload the collective and individual burdens that have weighed on our health. Please look at the Hermes Protocol with a deeper *"understanding."* Not cursory skimming. There is no shortcut "answer." In fact, I know of only one treatment for Genital Herpes that works 100% of the time. Not getting infected in the first place.

There's a HUGE shovel full of dirt (herpes trigger) coming down the mineshaft of my life. My wife just informed me she wants a divorce. She's scheduled a mediation hearing. I'll keep our progress posted throughout the book-writing process. It has merit, as it relates to the herpes stress factor.

July 28, 2017: as I'm about to retire for the evening, I glance at an ABC News http://bit.ly/2GqpgdeABCNews headline. Angelina Jolie is also struggling with divorce, as well as Bell's Palsy. It's an uncommon and puzzling (no, not divorce) neurologic condition that leads to one sided facial paralysis. Affected persons develop facial weakness in a matter of hours. Symptoms may include sagging facial eyebrows, a droop to the mouth, and unable to close the eye(s). Because of its physical abnormalities, people restrict many, if not most of their social interactions. Sounds a little like HSV. *"Gee, that's too bad,"* you're saying, but what does Bell's Palsy have to do with herpes? Risk factors for Bell's Palsy include pregnancy, diabetes, immune deficiency, and *yes*, the **Herpes Simplex Virus.**

The exact cause of Bell's Palsy is unknown. Scientists believe there is a link between inflammation and the reactivation of a dormant viral infection that affects the facial nerves. *"In most cases, symptoms resolve completely. However, people who do not have some recovery within 21 days have a greater risk of lasting facial muscle weakness."* Conventional treatment includes prednisone and antiviral medications such as Acyclovir. On rare occasions, surgery is needed to help relieve symptoms. LifeExtension.com has an excellent protocol that includes dietary, lifestyle, and integrative interventions that may also help. http://bit.ly/2Bzi9M1Palsy.

C. Health Crisis

Living sick and dying young in affluent America. Despite shelling out more money on healthcare than any other country in the world, almost half of all American adults have at least one chronic health disorder. And it's not just Americans getting sicker, it's young Americans that are unwell. A report by the National Research Council and Institute of Medicine (NRC/IOM) confirmed the gravity of its findings. Americans have been dying at younger ages than almost all other high-income countries. http://bit.ly/2FogrzmNRC

Industrialized medicine today is automated. Doctors increasingly treat lab results, x-rays, and blood pressure readings. Patient care and quality has deteriorated. For example, physicians spend on average 27% of their workday with patients, while more than 50% percent on Electronic Health Records (EHRs) and deskwork. And if that wasn't enough, another two hours of their personal time is "catching up" on paperwork.

Even though more-and-more of us are chronically sick and immune compromised, medicine's battle cry remains the same. *"We're the real doctors; down with quacks."* Directed at anyone who uses natural medicine and doesn't follow their *"outdated"* rules:

1. Go to our schools,
2. Get the licenses we control,
3. Don't make waves, and
4. Never deviate from the *"Standard of Care."*

Individual Americans aren't the only ones facing a health crisis and financial concerns. In 2017 the State of Illinois went *"from horrific financial health, to catastrophic, to broken."* Because of our failed *"sick-care"* system, the courts ordered the state to pay $586,000,000 million per month to catch up on their unpaid Medicaid bills. That's not a misprint. They were ordered to pay half a billion dollars per month just to catch up.

Wait a minute! *Do you mean to say that medicine is about profit, a return on investment, and earnings?* Yes, I suspect there is a conspiracy both in Congress and the FDA, and for good measures you might as well include medical boards. They want to *"criminalize natural and safe medicines,"* while pushing for high-priced prescription drugs. Public institutions like Illinois are crumbling under the burden of monopoly-priced medicine. *"Sick-care"* in America is a little bit like a *"legal drug cartel. A profiteering monopoly that transfers economic wealth from citizens to the pockets of drug companies."* Like the proverbial needle in the haystack, health, like herpes, is often difficult to find after it's been lost, until it accidentally *sticks* to us. *Congratulations!* Keep sticking to reading, even though the **Hermes Protocol** is not a needle, but a compass. And like any good compass, its purpose is to guide us back to well-being and happiness.

D. Orthodox or Alternative

Orthodox medicine values statistics and randomized double-blind clinical studies, which is OK if studying a single drug like Valtrex, or a specific surgical treatment, but it snubs its nose at more complex protocols of healing. Multipart components interact and work synergistically and are difficult to control, like herpes, people, and social media.

A good example of orthodox medicine's approach is to read any medication insert found in every drug container. Most seems written in Latin, with ambiguous terminology, lopsided comparisons, and unclear statistics. Even after years of complaints, they are still a big disappointment. Poorly written, overly technical, I've never finished reading one.

Medicine also has a long history of trying to discredit the truth about alternative treatments, yet more-and-more people are choosing a natural approach. Medicine's primary focus remains on crisis intervention and avoids examining its failure treating chronic diseases with symptom suppression.

Patients function with suppressive *"symptom"* therapy, but like caffeine, they often require an ever-increasing dose. Or the drugs stop working altogether. The next phase in the disease process is surgery by removing whatever isn't working. And the infection continues to pick up speed. *"Anti-herpetic agents reduce recurrence of herpes simplex-2 (HSV-2) symptoms but do not completely block subclinical shedding of virus, even at high doses, researchers reported."* http://bit.ly/2nINgXdHSV2 I've often wondered why our immune system fails to keep herpes or any disease dormant? **Dr. Max Gerson** believed our system's failure was due to the decline of our defenses brought about by:

1. Mineral and vitamin deficiency.
2. Toxins in the food supply from damaged soil.
3. The overuse of pesticides and fungicides.
4. Use of hormones found in animals we consume.
5. Eating processed, sugar-laden foods, and using
6. Alcohol, cigarettes, and street or prescribed drugs

Many people would rather take a pill, a shot, have surgery, and continue living a damaged lifestyle, rather than change their ways. What people don't understand is that we can stop breaking down our bodies at any time. **Dr. Max Gerson** believed they are not willing to change their situation until, *"the knife is at their throat,"* or Bell's Palsy, or Eczema Herpeticum. Not all disease states are lifestyle related. Other factors could be responsible:

1. Heredity.
2. Damaged immune system from birth.
3. Disease states from overuse of antibiotics.
4. Overexposure to pesticides while in utero.
5. Underarm deodorants containing aluminum, and
6. An altered immune system that attacks the body.

CAUTION: No food-processing chemical or pesticide treatment is safe. As the body accumulates toxins, we compound the problem by nourishing it with processed food grown from artificially fertilized soils. Eventually we lose our immunity and defenses.

E. Birth of Herpes

The Greek god, Apollo, was the Archer and god of healing. He healed the sick, but also brought out disease and plagues in man. Not much different from our immune system. It can either trigger or prevent herpes. *"I'm sorry, all your tests are normal, there's nothing more we can do for you. Either take this drug or learn to live with it."* After walking out of the doctor's office, I looked with dread at the Acyclovir Rx script, knowing its side effects, and then only getting partial relief.

The Gift that Keeps on Giving: a long, long time ago, Zeus sent Pandora (which means all-gifts) down to earth. She carried with her a small box with a big lock. It was a present for Epimetheus. When Zeus gave Epimetheus the key, he advised him to marry Pandora. But at the same time, he warned him, *"Never let anyone open the box!"*

Even though Pandora pleaded with him day after day to let her look inside the box, he always refused. Until one shadow-less sunrise. In darkness, Pandora's curiosity prevailed over her developed judgment. She pinched the key from under Epimetheus pillow and opened the box.

"Screeeckkk... eeekkk...," out flew untold suffering. Forces of terror that man never knew existed. Like locusts, swarms of misfortune took flight: sickness, disease, hate, betrayal, and the dreaded eternal **Herpesviridae.** They scattered into the fields of human discord. Pandora wept and tried to catch and put the cruel things back. But it was too late. The forces of misery had scattered, and herpes was free to roam the nerves of darkness. As Pandora lamented, she noticed the very last thing to fly out. It was not as sinister or painful looking like the others. And it turned out to be mankind's most human condition—**hope.** Zeus knew beforehand that hope would be needed when *"complicated problems arise out of unwise interference."*

If you've been affected or infected by herpes, specialness, or *"unwise interference,"* and life feels like living in *"a small box with a big lock."* Or uttered *"why me?"* or "but you-don't-understand," this book may help change the course of your Pandora life.

Hermes the Greek Messenger god: in Homer's Odyssey, Hermes healed the god Odysseus. Myth has it, *"All of us here, who are suffering..., need the help of Hermes if we are to get out."* The Hermes Protocol is designed to facilitate that process.

Herpes is a DNA virus that replicates in the nucleus of our cells. The blisters are its physical symptoms. According to Stanford University, the virus has been around since the Grecian time of Hermes. It is one of the oldest sexually transmitted infections (STIs) known to man, documented, and treated with limited success for thousands of years. http://stanford.io/2FoKxT5

The father of medicine, Hippocrates (460 to 370 BC), wrote about herpes lesions and their symptoms. Later, the Roman Emperor, Tiberius tried to quell an oral herpes outbreak by banning kissing at public celebrations. And the Roman physician, Celsus developed a treatment that cauterized open herpes lesions with a hot iron. It is believed that Shakespeare also mentioned herpes in Romeo and Juliet: *"O'er ladies lips. Which oft the angry Mab with 'blisters-plagues' because their breaths with sweetmeats tainted are. Act 1. Scene IV"* And the *"quest"* continues.

F. Jokes, Scams, and Myths

*"**Genital Herpes** is mostly a magnet for jokes, scams, and myths."* When I first read that line, I thought they were talking about some other *"nastiness."* Maybe rotten crotch (most likely fungus), or *"My Boner ist Kaput"* (Erectile Dysfunction), or stinky, squishy, and proud (Incontinence), but not Genital Herpes.

Genital Herpes is a virus, not good or bad, right, or wrong, moral, or immoral, etc., or etc. Herpes only feels impure because we've managed to coat it with a puritanical, sexual patina that wears a Frankenstein mask. But it's seldom fatal and less benign than most diseases. Women remain its immoral targets and victims. The *"stakes"* have not changed. It still burns. Tied to posts and tweets of late night one liners, and religious blistery retributions, is it any wonder that women feel wounded, depressed, betrayed, angry, and resentful? Herpetic sex between consenting adults is fraught enough with trials and frustrations. Making it an opening punch line for every talk show, or Fake News Network, only exasperates the gift that keeps on giving.

Herpes is not a coincidence: it's our canary in a world of pain. Before trying to put it back into Pandora's box, first wrap it in forgiveness. If that doesn't work, get even. Sleep with them. You can tell I'm a bit burned-out by the *"I'm not much, but it's all I think about"* Holly-woo-woo-better-than-you-you-crowd. If herpes wasn't so painful and stressful, it would almost be worth having again. I could become a predator and fever-blister their mouths shut. *"Oh, I'm sorry for calling you stupid and insensitive. I thought you knew."*

So, what are the *Holy-woo-woos* doing to eliminate the stigma and shame surrounding Genital Herpes? http://bit.ly/2Gqr59RSTIGMA In a word. **Nothing**. They're too busy *Weinsteining*. In the past, celebrities often used their status to help raise awareness for health issues. On occasion they even opened-up about their own disease. Cancer, lupus, diabetes, and even HIV. But to date, no *woo-woo* has come forward and admitted being infected with Genital Herpes. Or stepped up to help eliminate its stigma. That doesn't stop the tabloids from spitting out their names about which stars have herpes or STDs.

"I-Me-Me-I-Me-Crowd" can't help it. They've been infected with that rare *HSV-I-Me-Me-6ex* mutation that doesn't break out in blisters, but *"blusters"* endless vitriolic verbal disdain and condemnation of everyone and everything (pretty much like I'm doing now). I wonder if I caught it hugging' some *"love-ya"* Woo-Woo at Hollywood's Chinese Grumman's Theater. Think about it. Every time we open an app, flip channels, watch NBA Basketball or Ding-Dong-CNN, diabolical Jack from *The Shining*, pops-up playing news anchor. *"Here's Johnny,"* doing some hostile, blistery commentary on another Zika health care crisis. *"Yikes!"* From Johnny's crazed look, he may be sitting on a Zika. *"Better ask your doctor!"*

Yes, we live in a burned-out, social-media driven world. Bought, polluted, infected, or modified to suit special interests. How many pharmaceutical advertisements do you watch and then make an appointment to *"ask your doctor?"* Perhaps some of the TV *"Woo-Woos"* don't have breakouts. But they sure sound burned out. Exhausted, without perspective, depressed, and internally empty. They offer little more than condemnation, while condoning everything and everyone. Maybe it takes the focus off their own *Weltschmerz*. What about a solution that doesn't speak to special interest?

This brings up a point that will be repeated throughout the **Hermes Protocol.** Be gentle with yourself while healing from Genital Herpes. It is not an *"on-and-off"* switch, but a process. With the Hermes Protocol it will get better. First, in an unpleasant way. There are lifestyle, supplement, and mental changes that can initially cause tension. Please, try not to criticize, judge, or blame yourself or anyone else through mental, verbal, or social-media thoughts, texts, tweets, or messages. Stay mindful. By not accusing or attacking, our fear and anger is diminished. We become less afraid. Hermes Protocol has two methods in working with the mind and its thoughts. With practice, they will change how you perceive yourself and the world.

In the Biblical world, the number seven (7) stood for wholeness. A six (6) meant you were *"short of being the real thing."* So how does someone regain their balance (Number 7) and recover from herpes burnout (Number 6)? It's quite simple, you add one to six. I wish it were that simple. Although not rocket science, it's a bit more complex.

I was your typical herpes blame-and-prey victim poster child. Tried to escape from my own body, looking to be rescued, nurtured, and/or understood by my significant other. Water under the vows. Exhausted, I made peace with the enemy and climbed out of the valley of dis-ease and self-absorption. Try to remember, when sad, bitter, resentful, and angry: *"Our partners will not be able to rescue us from our own life."* Or even understand the pain, depression, frustration, or panic attacks we experience. Few will comprehend what we're going through. Unless you're unfortunate or fortunate enough to have another herpes sufferer in your life.

G. Out of Love

*"Raise your words, not voice.
It is rain that grows flowers, not thunder."* – Rumi

In life's unpredictable journey, Genital Herpes often separates us from loved ones. If herpes gets between you, don't let outbreaks isolate you. We can help each other. Email rhermes1@gmail.com with your phone number and the best time to call you. A brief description of questions or issues. I'll get back to you as soon as I can.

Eczema Herpeticum played a part in losing my marriage. Like any health crisis that demands our constant attention, it's a price many of us pay when we're challenged with a chronic disease. But working with the Hermes Protocol, we re-discover who we are. Feelings of loneliness, grief, and guilt turn into appreciation, self-worth, and contentment. It also helped writing the Hermes Protocol when I realized Genital Herpes is not as important as helping others.

Of all the books I've read, or movies seen, none has ever approached the feelings of awe and wonder of *"falling in love,"* or despair of falling out. But then none of my media heroes ever confessed to Genital Herpes. As pervasive as it is, it might be a good idea to start including it in marriage vows. *"In herpes dormancy, and in breakouts, until infections do us part."* Chronic herpes infections have a way of unmasking what many dread most, they're unlovable. During an active outbreak, herpes background chatter can sound like a Greek tragedy. *"I'm just not lucky in love,"* or *"I'm too damaged to love,"* or *"I'm through with love."*

Our Mask of Cynicism is there to hide the heartbreak of loneliness. In those wounded moments, a walled heart can seem like the best defense. But before giving up and rejecting love as a personal illusion, feeling it takes more than it gives, finish the Hermes Protocol. In some ways, committed relationships are like Genital Herpes. They break out in distress occasionally but then recede back into quiet dormancy. But not all. Some break out in chronic bickering, betrayal, and disappointments, ending up in therapy, mediation and/or asking their doctor for medication.

Questions Remain: how do we do this thing called life with a chronic disease like herpes? How to keep a better perspective? And then I remembered one of Mark Twain's words of wisdom. *"Kindness is the language which the deaf can hear, and the blind can see."* And in an *"Aha-Moment"* I realized the way to do *"It"* is without Clinging or Controlling (C&C).

Clinging and Controlling: feels different then *"letting go and letting be."* C&C is holding on too long, mentally always wanting more. Whether at the gym, clutching heavy luggage, "clinging" from a tree branch, or coveting that brand-new F-150. Sooner than later our muscles, nervous system, checkbook, and mind get fatigued. We're forced to let go because we can't afford that vacation or truck. However, letting go or detaching doesn't mean we're not involved or present. It's just that we're not trying to control **People, Places, and Things (PPT)**. The more we try to hold on or manage PPT, the more distress, suffering, and unhappiness we live through.

Words of caution: letting go doesn't mean getting rid of, dropping out, disliking certain people or situations, and dodging them. That's not letting go, but a form of avoidance. We enhance our letting go, by thinking of it as ***"letting be."*** Have you noticed these days that casual interactions amongst friends, or even family members, can quickly turn into disagreements and then full-blown arguments? Someone's insensitive social media post upsets people to where they block or cut ties forever. Like a divorce, but without a marriage certificate to burn because of irreconcilable differences.

Not only COVID-19 or Herpes: but life in general is more disruptive and isolating. Increasingly, people shy away from social settings, avoid light-hearted conversations, preferring the companionship of their iPhones for *"cuddling."* Yes, COVID or Genital Herpes can make *"outbreak inmates"* of us. But they are not alone. It's a phenomenon today that is common throughout society. We are more separated and isolated.

"Opposing points of view on women's rights, gay marriage, immigration, human rights, family values, foreign relations, politics, and religion (just to name a few), with surprising frequency are driving wedges and creating conflict between friends and family. It seems as if everyone is either with 'us or them.' In which case "them-others" violate our sense of what's right, fair, and good. How do you stand up for what's right or stand against what's wrong without putting more opposition, negativity, fear, and separation into the world?"
Eckhart Tolle

Genital Herpes: is only one of countless reasons for the collapse of many traditional social interactions and values. Blasted with a constant barrage of COVID negativity and fear mongering from the media, we compound the problem by avoidance and escaping vis-a-vis our addictive quest for *"more-and-more"* pleasure instead of seeking real and lasting happiness. There are simple ways to achieve happiness that are free, opposed to fleeting pleasures that often carry a steep price tag of addiction and despair.

Genital Herpes can affect every aspect of life. Whether single, married, or in a committed relationship, each person responds to herpes in their own way, depending on their experience with illness, familial history, personal values, psychological makeup, finances, or health insurance. Or whether they live alone or a couple. Often, one person's emotional quicksand will be another's greatest act of bravery. While herpetic infections often raise questions and issues for the infected person. Partners are also faced with their own challenges. Depending on the frequency and severity of outbreaks, unwelcome thoughts can creep into a partner's consciousness.

1. *"Should I stay or cut my losses and go?"*
2. *"What about our sex life?"*
3. *"What do I do when there isn't any?"*
4. *"Then what happens to our intimacy?"*
5. *"Will our relationship ever feel the same again?"*
6. *"I'm scared that I might get infected."*

When diagnosed with Genital Herpes most people are forced to navigate through unchartered territory. Not only with medical uncertainty but coming to terms with a current or future relationship. If in a committed relationship, you might be staring into a foggy future of solitude. There is anguish in losing spontaneous intimacy. It will test the level of your resilience with the person you love most. Or examine the shallowness of forgiveness in yourself or your partner.

Love between two people is never simple, but none more complicated than when there is a third party like COVID-19 or **Genital Herpes.** We pretend to know what love is. Seldom acknowledging how powerful and lasting its currents are. We expect it to be healing and whole, even when faced with a chronic disease. Then we are astonished to find that love at times is frail and human, affecting division in relationships and failures in marriages. Plato said that *"love is a kind of madness, a divine madness."* His point was that when we fall in love, most of us don't think. In fact, our reasoning takes a back seat. Bouncing between, *"joy, exhilaration, euphoria, increased energy, sleeplessness, loss of appetite, trembling, a racing heart, and accelerated breathing, or anxiety, panic, and feelings of despair,"* at the slightest hint that our *"special"* relationship has flaws.

We tend to focus on the positive, drowning out any danger signs. And like any good addict, we'll do just about anything to make sure our mounting passion of romance and chemistry will be forever by our side, including getting married or *"until death do us part."* Researchers say that being in love is a form of addiction. And like most addicts, we'll make promises that are challenging, if not impossible to keep. Then to make matters worse, we not only promise but *"vow"* before God to love and honor each other *"for better or for worse, in herpes-hell or in glowing-health."*

Question? Would you marry the love of your life if they were breaking out with Genital Herpes every 10 days? What's the cut-off? What kind of honeymoon lovefest are we talking about? It never occurred to me or my wife *"for worse"* or *"in sickness"* would turn into an outbreak emotional roller-coaster marathon, including a nasty Eczema Herpeticum steeplechase. Knowing what we know today, I'm sure neither would've committed to such an ordeal. But then the *"for worse"* only happens to the *"others"* on the 6 o'clock news, not us decent folks.

Life doesn't always go according to our illusions. One day, within our mundane turbulence of going to work, coming home and grocery shopping, balancing an overdrawn checkbook, and doing a week's worth of laundry, something happens that you didn't count on. You have a Genital Herpes outbreak. Then another, and another. And they keep coming. In 2022 you're just relieved it's not COVID-19. For most, Genital Herpes breaks out without warning, then disappears and goes back into hibernation, seldom to be heard from again. But for a few, to test their promises or vows, an occurrence turns into a marathon of complicated skin rashes, headaches, tiredness, confusion, and an unfamiliar reaction that has your doctor concerned.

For Couples: nonstop herpes infections are not just a diversion of single solitaire, but a 24-7 game of war. Without any victor. When one partner is infected, both lives are interrupted. Like any chronic illness, Genital Herpes outbreaks disrupt day-to-day routines and life's familiar patterns. It forces relationships to dig deeper. Many times, to their bedrock, having to make decisions that were unthinkable just a year prior. It's never easy. As a result, some couples fall and break apart. Others decide to stay together but are forced into assuming different responsibilities and roles. The honeymoon is over. *By the way "Mr. Herpes or is it Hermes? I had my fingers crossed when I spoke those vows."*

No single therapeutic approach for Genital Herpes is one-hundred percent (100%) **right** for everyone. If it were, you'd already be doing it. Each person responds to herpes and its management in their own unique way. The choices we make, whether to use alternative protocols or orthodox medicine, are influenced by many different biological, emotional, and mental factors. Including your past medical history, social mores, personal values, psychological makeup, finances, and determination to follow through with a chosen treatment. They will all influence your outcome.

The process is easier with a strong supportive partner, rather than being in the late stages of a tired, weathered relationship. But statistics or demographics seldom determine who gets well and who continues to suffer. If we recover from chronic herpes infections, it's usually not without repairing our immune system and restless mind.

Churchill said, *"Those that fail to learn from history are doomed to repeat it"*? I like my version better: *"History repeats itself because no one ever listens."* What used to be the bedrock of every *"traditional"* marriage are the wedding vows. They are words we speak to each other which express both *"an intent and a promise."* It provides a relationship through which husband and wife support each other.

Our marriage is 'kaput,' and we're in the divorce Fast-Tract-Carpool lane. Our vows did not save us, and I know from my first divorce; it can be a long and painful process that never seems to end. And we're never quite sure if we've done the right thing. Even if there is some peace of mind about our decision, memories and attachments continue to persist, even if only in our subconsciousness. Genital Herpes is only too glad to *breakout and join* the stress party our mind is throwing.

***Auf-wiedersehen* marriage, hello herpes.** Repetitive Genital Herpes infections are like a troubled marriage. The never-ending arguments that break out, without knowing what triggers them, or how to stop them. The key to change in any relationship is commitment. To accept and to let go and let be. That doesn't mean we don't work on issues, or adjust our attitude, but we must be willing to stay and not flee from conflict. Sometimes change happens not because we've decided to be nicer or act in a more compassionate way, but because all relationships and marriages have cracks, and eventually, that's how the light shines in. With light, we gain a better perspective.

What do you expect? Some relationships fall apart, no matter what you do. Don't think it's his or her fault. It's just life. Before you get into any relationship, please read the fine print of the marriage certificate. It might work, or it might not. But no matter what happens, we can learn and grow from our experience. Whichever way it goes, we don't blame anyone. If it works, great. If it doesn't, that's okay, too. We learn more from things falling apart than staying together. The fallen *"parts"* turn into wisdom *fertilizer* for growing more conscious and spiritual. This is how we grow up and learn to be more compassionate, the building blocks for a more peaceful life. If things only went well or our way, we wouldn't be able to grow into the kind of caring and forgiving person we want to be. Our difficulties and misfortunes nourish our wisdom, making us more compassionate and forgiving.

Relationships are unpredictable. The more time and distance we have in life, the more we realize some couples stay together, while others fall apart and get divorced. It's nobody's fault, only a learning period for both partners. Therefore, it can also be a mutually positive experience. Yes, there may be grief and pain, but only because we want to cling and hang on to something that's no longer there.

There is never any justification for revenge or anger. No matter what the other person did or didn't do. We accept them and move on. That's the only way we'll ever change in a positive way and have any chance of future happiness. This is often a difficult concept to accept. We're so used to seeing the world through our *"justified-revenge"* bifocals. Black or white, right, or wrong, and good or bad. But like pleasure, it doesn't lead to happiness.

My Marriage was like a *"good ol' Western."* Characters came and went across the screen of life's open West. The hero rides into town and falls in love with Kitty, the local saloon girl. They got married and raised a life together on a small ranch. But one day we see the saloon girl in a stagecoach, alone with their children, leaving the cowhand in the dust. There was no awakening for Kitty or the cowboy.

We are left feeling alone. Much the same way we are born and die alone. In between there is an opportunity to overcome and transcend our aloneness and connect with others. But no matter how good or long the marriage or movie lasts, eventually it must end. Just like all relationships ultimately end. Whether through divorce or a partner dies. The movie has ended. The good news, there's always another movie coming out next week. Let's wait and see if our cowboy is still riding alone, or if Kitty is serving up a nice-cold brewski to our new hero. Well, maybe not ice cold. It was the wild West without refrigeration. The show has ended but try not to blame yourself or Genital Herpes.

Advocates of Love: dependable relationships are built on strong spiritual foundations, reinforced by five characteristics to strengthen, and embrace their success:

1. **Commitment**
2. **Forgiveness**
3. **Trust**
4. **Respect**
5. **The Now**

First Advocate: Commitment

Talk less and do more. Show your commitment to relationships through actions. If a partner has Genital Herpes, learn about Genital Herpes to show your support. When we don't feel commitment from our partners, it's difficult to feel love if devotion is lacking. Clouded by nonstop stress from chronic herpes outbreaks, it'll be a matter of time before the relationship implodes. Recognize this dilemma or separation is imminent.

Second Advocate: Forgiveness

Forgiveness does not ignore the truth of Genital Herpes suffering. Forgiveness is not weak. It calls for courage and integrity. Forgiveness and love can bring about the peace we long for. *"True love is not for the faint-hearted."* All of us have hurt and betrayed others, just as they've harmed us. Extending and receiving forgiveness is essential for redemption from our past. To forgive does not mean we condone the wrongs of others. *"Forgiveness means giving up all hope for a better past."* It's a way to move on.

How do we forgive someone who infected us with Genital Herpes? A partner who lied. Or put aside betrayals in a relationship? And most of all, how can we forgive ourselves? Discover something in your partner or another that's worthy of respect. Once realized, that *"something"* can become the spark or match to light the fire of forgiveness. Feelings of revenge, guilt, and anger surface when we see nothing in the person or relationship worth saving. With this approach, like the hand in front of our eyes, we've lost perspective. Our partners are never quite as bad as we make them out to be. If there is something worth saving and respecting, then the relationship can be revived.

How to ask for forgiveness. Out of my hurt and anger, fear, and confusion, I realize how I've hurt you. Caused you much discomfort by infecting you with herpes. So, I want to take this moment to ask for your forgiveness. *"Please forgive me. Can you see it in your heart to forgive me? If so, thank you."*

How to forgive ourselves. Completing the circle of forgiveness. While my heart remains open, I also want to be compassionate and extend forgiveness to myself. While looking into the mirror, *"I hold myself with forgiveness and mercy. I forgive myself for not having been more careful with my herpes infection, and not a better, more honest partner."* And gently, I repeat, *"I forgive myself."*

How to forgive others. We've all been betrayed and hurt. It's not easy to forget the pain and heartache of Genital Herpes infections. But to the degree that I'm ready, I'm willing to turn my heart in the direction of forgiveness, and to the extent that I'm able to forgive you for infecting me with herpes, *"I forgive you. I offer you forgiveness, and I release you. I will not carry the pain or bitterness in my heart."* And even though I don't feel lightness, I'm prepared to do the

Life without forgiveness would be unbearable. Like politics, we would be chained to the suffering of our past. Repeating it over and over again without release or relief. To love and forgive is not for the faint hearted. But somehow, we must step up and say, it stops with me. *"I will accept and bear the suffering, but I will not retaliate."*

Forgiveness is not so much about Genital Herpes, or the other person, nor is it sentimental. It's a deep reflection on the hurt, anger, and fear in our hearts. To let it open and release its pain. As the heart is pulled apart, grief pours out. A natural process of the loss we experienced being infected with Genital Herpes. Life didn't work out as planned. What's that saying one more time?

"Forgiveness is giving up all hope for a better past."

Forgiveness is seldom quick. It can take time. It's also not sentimental, condoning, or papering over our pain. But most of all, it's not for anyone else but ourselves. We see the benefits of a loving heart. Recognize it's not necessary to be loyal to our herpetic suffering or the drama it entails. *"What happened to me? The betrayal is about me. Me, me, me… OK, OK, OK, enough ego, calm down."* The Genital Herpes infection happened. Yes, my partner left. Yes, it's horrible. And yes, I'm still doing *"healing-work."* But the pain and heartache does not define who I am. I choose to live in peace and joy, even amongst those who ostracize and shame the infected. In peace, even amongst those who blame.

"Don't reject your grief and loneliness,
let it season you like no ingredients can." -Rumi

Everybody who loves suffers loss in some way. Why should those with herpes be any different? Be grateful for the grief; otherwise, we would never experience the feeling of love. Remember, the pursuit of happiness does not mean the *"right to happiness."* Happiness is a worthwhile endeavor, but there is something even more profound and joyful. Stay tuned.

Third Advocate: Trust
Trust is love. The demons of jealousy, fear, anger, control, and guilt are the thugs that rob us of our faith. They undermine the love in any relationship. But no one betrays our trust more than ourselves. If you've misplaced trust, *"Rest in Peace,"* and realize you are not a *"self-made man (or woman) who worships their creator."* That only works if you live alone or are institutionalized. We will help you find your trust if you've lost it.

Fourth Advocate: Respect
It begins with self-respect and then expands outward toward our partners and others. To respect our partner means that in our eyes they are someone we can look up to. If respect and appreciation turn to disregard and disapproval, the relationship suffers. In time it breaks down. Appreciating the other person's unique talents creates respect. Without it we sink into criticism and nitpicking before separating.

Fifth Advocate: The Now
Most eyes are turned toward the future. It's only in the *here-and-now* that relationships grow in love. Yes, hope can temporarily salvage a relationship by planning to create a better future. But it's in the *Now* that we feel love. Why? Because that's all there ever is. There is only ever the *Now*. The future and past are the ego's stranglehold on our contentment. Unhappy people are seldom *in the moment*. They're reflecting on their past *"herpetic"* mistakes or their future *"outbreak"* uncertainty.

When unhappy people get into relationships, they're happy for about a week, because they're not thinking about the future or past. Then, things get ordinary again. That happiness relationship mirage vanishes into the horizon of fear and foreboding unease. *If only I had this or that, or didn't have those, then I'd be happy.* Most of us know that's NOT true, but we buy into it. It's NOT out there! Anywhere.

I'll leave you with this thought about relationship and herpes. Many things in life can be fixed. Herpes may be one of them. But many times, relationships between two people cannot be fixed. Because they should not be fixed. Create something out of Genital Herpes, **"My Friend, the Enemy,"** experience, even if your relationship falls apart make use of it. Try not to buy into the ego's fantasy that once you *"find the perfect partner everything will be OK."* It's the same belief over-and-over again that once I change my *"situation,"* quit my job, exchange my husband, live by myself, and be Genital Herpes free, then I'll be happy. Good luck. Email me after a couple of months and let me know how well that's working for you. The truth resides in the *"Now."*

PART TWO: HERPES LIFE CYCLE

From Host to Hostage

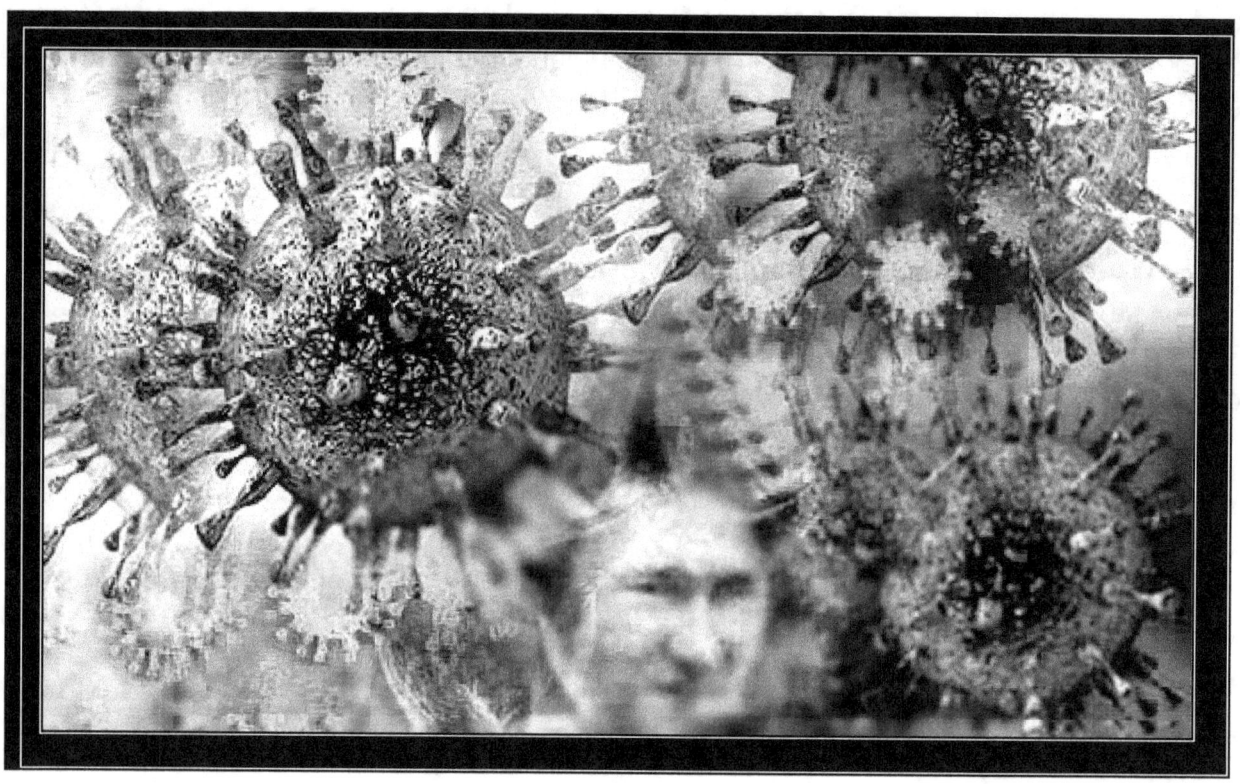

Chapter 3: Herpes

The Good, Bad, Technical: according to Wikipedia http://bit.ly/2DVWCIWiki, *"Herpesviridae"* is a large family of DNA viruses, (herpesviruses) derived from the Greek word *herpein* or *"to creep."* As in recurring outbreaks or infections give me the *"creeps."* In total, there are about 130 herpes viruses. Most are found in mammals, birds, fish, reptiles, amphibians, and mollusks. Depending on your source, 90% of U.S. adults are infected with at least one of the following:

1. **HSV-1**, infections often occur around the mouth, lips, nose, or face.
2. **HSV-2**, infections can involve the labia, genitals, sacrum, buttocks, and anus.
3. **Varicella Zoster** virus, the cause of chickenpox and shingles.
4. **Epstein-Barr** virus, implicated in mononucleosis and some cancers.
5. **Cytomegalovirus**, and
6. **Human papillomavirus** (HPV).

Researching herpes statistics on the Internet you might come to two conclusions. Either nobody knows what they're talking about, or nobody really knows. Not because the research is flawed, but because individuals get confused communicating statistics. They keep trying to fit their definition of HSV into science and research. That's why the CDC recently added a comment on its Genital Herpes page: **http://bit.ly/2FoogoACDC** *"The overall prevalence of Genital Herpes (HSV-2) is likely higher than 16.2%, because an increasing number of Genital Herpes infections are caused by HSV-1. Increases in genital HSV-1 infections have been found in patient populations worldwide."* A bigger problem than herpes statistics, most people (85%) don't know they're infected. They've never been symptomatic.

How do You Prevent: getting infected with HSV? It's difficult. Human beings make human contact. There are steps we can take to reduce the risk, but at some point, somewhere, by someone, nearly everyone gets infected. **So, what's the good news?** Over 80% tolerate HSV just fine. This book may not be for them, although the Hermes Protocol is for anyone who wants to enjoy better health. For the 20% who suffer, and whose lives are compromised by chronic Genital Herpes infections, stay tuned. Although this book is about herpes, the Human Papillomavirus Virus (HPV) is the most common sexually transmitted infection. Most sexually active men and women are exposed to it at some point. http://bit.ly/2DIgSUPHPV

To Prevent: the spread of **Genital Herpes,** avoid all sexual contact during an outbreak. Always use condoms. It's not a guarantee, just like an auto umbrella insurance policy is not a guarantee against getting into an accident. But no matter what, don't drive your stick shift without a condom. It doesn't matter whether you're infected with HSV-1 or HSV-2, the **Hermes Protocol** is effective for both. The contamination risk for the other partner is the same. Anyone infected with HSV of either type can transmit HSV to their partner at any time if those parts make contact.

Statistics Does Not diminish fear. The average number of sexual encounters is about two dozen (24) *"love-ins"* before being infected with Genital Herpes. The number seems inflated because Herpes doesn't live on the skin's surface, but in our nerve endings. The predator hides out until it randomly emerges into the skin for transmission. With or without an outbreak. However, during an active outbreak there are far more viruses available to infect a partner. So, it's best to avoid sex during that time. Considering herpes prevalence, we could acquire it from just about anyone. Even as far back as years ago. The irony? Most of us are already infected. We may not know it.

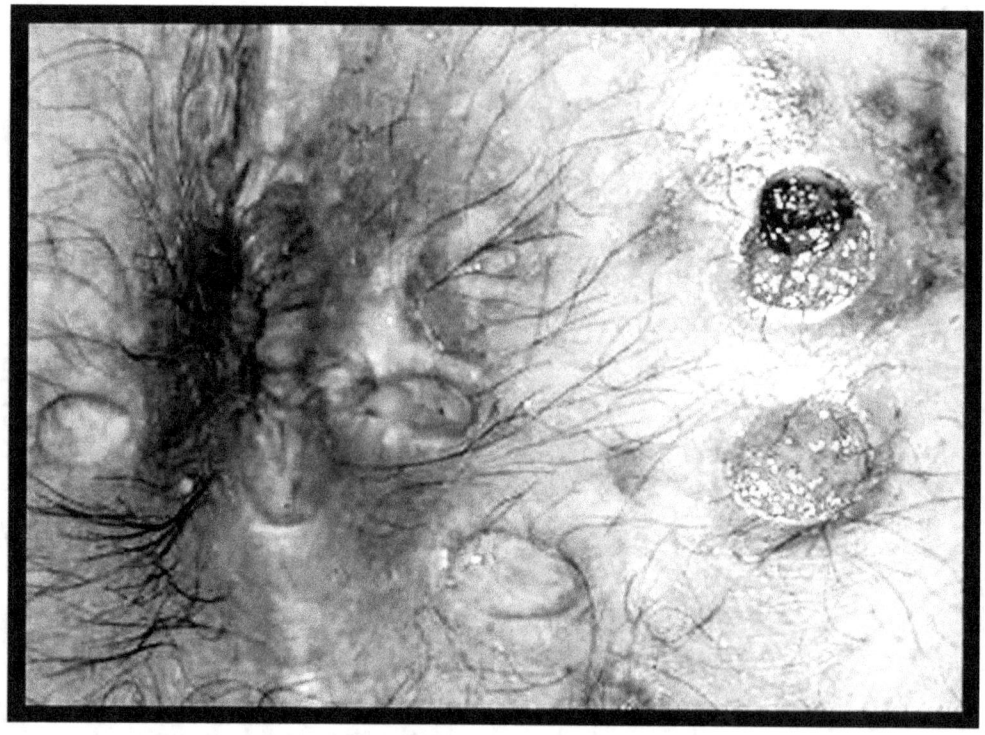

Sacral Herpes before the Hermes Protocol

During the initial infection, the herpes virus replicates in cell after cell at the point of origin. Like any living organism, its purpose is to reproduce and spread. Immediately, the immune system responds. A fierce battle starts, which can manifest itself as an *"outbreak."* Herpes functions by taking over a living cell. That cell becomes a viral host. To deactivate the virus, our immune system kills the cell and the virus. Like guerilla warfare, the herpes virus escapes the immune system by traveling up nerve fibers to an area known as ganglia. In effect, it hides out, and viral replication ceases. Herpes is then considered *"dormant."*

***"Darth"* Herpes** uses *"Star-Wars"* cloaking maneuvers to avoid discovery and demise. The immune system can't "see" the virus while it's dormant. For those with strong and vigilant immune system, herpes can stay hidden for years, then appear when we're *"run-down"* or immune compromised. Those with healthy immune systems often don't know they're infected.

Initial Symptoms: whether **HSV-2** or **HSV-1**, Genital Herpes indicators are not much different from those of cold sores. They can differ from person to person but are more complex for females. Symptoms include:

1. **Blisters** on and around the genital area, rectum, inner thighs, and buttocks
2. **For women**, blister can arise in the cervix and discharge from the vagina.
3. **Flu-like symptoms,** fever, chills, exhaustion, shooting pains, muscle aches.
4. **Urinary Tract Infections (UTIs).**
5. **Pain** when urinating for both genders.
6. **Infections** normally last about two weeks.
7. **Doctors** generally treat HSV-2 with antiviral medication.

Please see your health care provider ASAP if you experience any rash or strange infection to *"test"* and make sure it's herpes.

A. Revenge of the Hippies

*"It is easier to fool people than to convince them
that they have been fooled."* – Mark Twain

Fifty years ago, young people from all over America came to San Francisco's Haight-Ashbury hoping to join the *"hippies,"* a new group of rebellious romantics that preached a life of peace, love, and happiness. It was the *"Summer-of-Love"* and a launch-pin for *"love-ins"* across America. The media was everywhere. *"Tabloid-news"* headlines launched a set of hippie myths that persist to this day. Similar to the COVID 'media' circus of today.

For us old wannabes, the sixties (1960s) re-kindled memories of the Beatles, Viet Nam, and of course, *"the hippies."* Even though hippies emerged from the sixties, they didn't hit their stride until the seventies (1970s). The same time **herpes** transformed from an *"alien"* into a *"happening."* In fact, doctors in the sixties (1960s) couldn't distinguish a cold sore from a genital sore. It was all just herpes. Outbreaks on your mouth or privates, were considered hippies. *"Oops, mainstream slip. I meant herpes."*

Herpes was below medicine's radar. So low that a standard medical textbook, *Obstetric and Gynecological Nursing* (Rosemary E Bailey, 1978 edition), didn't even list herpes in its index. A 1975 study of *"Psychological morbidity for sexually transmitted diseases,"* (Richard Mayou, The London Hospital) made no mention of Herpes. Today these exclusions are unthinkable. http://bit.ly/2DLTnhG

HSV Testing: began in the late '70s. By the '80s herpes changed from an itchy skin complaint, into a controversial viral infection. It wasn't long before the media gave birth to a *"good"* versus *"bad"* virus. Herpes on your mouth indicated appropriate behavior, while Genital Herpes signified *"hippie-free-love"* debauchery.

Just as HSV-1 and HSV-2 are two distinct viruses, the hippies separated into two diverse groups. The small, but vocal antiwar protesters, and those who embraced spiritual enlightenment and community building, along with sex, drugs, and rock-and-roll. One had little to do with the other. The more radicalized camp, like a feverish Genital Herpes outbreak, blended militant politics with hippie attire. The majority were non-violent, benevolent, easy-going. Like a mild cold sore. Indifferent to or opposed to any political activities. There were splinter groups. *The Brotherhood of Eternal Love*, from Laguna Beach, CA, used LSD as a path to enlightenment. It was LSD guru Dr. Timothy Leary who urged everyone to *"turn on, tune in, and drop out."* Meaning get high, disregard mainstream norms, look inward for peace and wisdom.

President Nixon called him the *"most dangerous virus in America."* (Oops, slipped up again.) The Laguna Beach police department confirmed that description by arresting him on January 21, 1970. Soon a lot more *"Brothers"* followed him to unawareness. Dr. Leary received a ten-year sentence for possession of two marijuana roaches. With an additional ten years added for a previous arrest for another marijuana possession. Twenty years to be served consecutively. Unlike herpes, Dr. Leary never broke out. But after serving six years, Governor Jerry Brown pardoned him.

To many an onlooker, the hippies were synonymous with *"free-lust."* Even though they were more adventuresome than main street, it was more hype than reality. Most headlines in tabloid journalism came from a few fanatical individuals. As one hippie recounted decades later, *"We had parties where people would smoke or drink too much and sleep with their friends, but there were emotional repercussions the next day. Free love is like a free lunch.* http://wapo.st/2nlwpTz *There's no such thing; even nudity was rare."*

In time, most *"love the one you're with"* enthusiasts of the 1960s and 1970s discovered the free-love-train was not a trouble-free ride. It also didn't take women long to realize that the sexual freedom of the hippie era didn't change their role. They just wore a different uniform. Tie-dyed costumes.

Sexually Transmitted

STIs and STDs are infections commonly spread from person to person through sexual contact. The acronyms are used interchangeably.

STD = Sexually Transmitted Disease
STI = Sexually Transmitted Infection

Religious 'sex-abstinence' advocates blamed the excesses of the sixties (1960s) for the rise of *"new"* STDs, such as **AIDS** and Genital Herpes. They asserted that syphilis and gonorrhea were the only STDs in existence until the 1960s. That, of course, isn't true. The hippies may have spread a lot of nastiness amongst themselves, but they didn't create the STD epidemic. Rates of syphilis and gonorrhea were so serious during World War I; our government mounted a nationwide campaign or faced a shortage of soldiers.

It's hard to believe that there was a time when *'Genital Herpes'* was not a stigmatized and feared condition. Both doctors and patients for the most part ignored it. The newly diagnosed were *not* made to feel like sexual-lepers or never having a chance at a meaningful relationship. Doctors back then simply dealt with and treated the common facial cold sore on a different site, the genitals or sacrum. Herpes was not invested with the fear that it commands today. The words *"Genital Herpes"* barely registered with the public. Except, of course, Officer Brezhnev.

The hippie fringe counterculture, with their love for yoga, organic food, and blue jeans, didn't *"die out."* Middle class America absorbed most of it as an accepted part of everyday life. Unlike the hippies, the herpes stigma of the eighties ('80s) remains.

By the 1960s, antibiotics had succeeded in healing the most feared bacterial STDs, like syphilis and gonorrhea. Pharmaceutical research then focused their efforts on the next Holy Grail, antiviral drugs. In the late 1970s, Burroughs Wellcome created a practical antiviral. With one small drawback. It only affected viruses in the herpes family: chickenpox and herpes simplex. And none of the conditions required treatment except in extreme cases. Almost everyone with a herpes infection recovered without treatment. The rest used topical solutions to ease the pain and manage healing. Three decades later, Dr. Pedro Cuatrecasas, who oversaw the R&D at Burroughs Wellcome from 1975 to 1985 said, "During the R&D of Acyclovir (Zovirax), the marketing department of Burroughs Wellcome insisted that there were 'no markets' for this compound. Most had never heard of Genital Herpes." http://bit.ly/2njUIky

Any public perception for the *need* for antiviral drugs would have to be manufactured. What do you know? Manufactured is an elaborate word for duping the public through marketing. It's also illegal in most countries. In fact, the United States and New Zealand are the only two countries that allow direct-to-consumer advertising of prescription drugs. Ever watched TV without a drug add stressing you to *"ask your doctor?"*

The answer to Burroughs' Acyclovir perception dilemma? Find a disease like the common cold that wasn't serious except on rare occasions. Yet make it 'potentially' risky to justify taking an expensive antiviral drug. Then make it seem even more dangerous to those who are not infected. *"Hello, stigma, goodbye herpes anonymity!"*

Boroughs' scandalous marketing motive was simple. They wanted a return on their investment. Their promotions were designed to stimulate demand for Acyclovir by raising concerns about the social consequences of a herpes infection and emphasizing that Acyclovir could reduce outbreaks and transmission. That their *"fear-mongering"* campaign was successful is like saying Mt. Everest is a tall mountain. They created a demand and stigma that has clung to our sacrum and lips ever since. Their "new" wonder drug ads were deceptive and misleading, and Genital Herpes acquired the status of an important and "risky" disease. Once the media noticed the word "incurable," meaning grave and hopeless, all bets were off. The stigma broke out and it's never healed. Herpes articles began to appear from *"Dear Abby"* to the cover story of *Time* magazine. Twice. Anything negative http://ti.me/2DIh8mA was over-dramatized to trigger more public concern.

The marketing of antiviral drugs has been one of the most successful "manufactured" examples of 'disease-mongering.' A process of exaggerating the consequence of a disease to increase sales. Like a bad fashion statement, everyone with an outbreak wanted an Acyclovir makeover. From that point on, the success of Acyclovir, Valtrex, and Famvir were guaranteed.

The Fallout from the Burroughs antiviral marketing campaign was not all gloom-and-doom. Acyclovir has provided many with serious Genital Herpes infections with more options and relief from various complications. And for that, I'm grateful. We don't question the integrity of the drug Acyclovir, only the motives and truthfulness of its manufacturer.

Herpes Stigma is not the same in all countries. In many non-English speaking countries, the word *'herpes'* translates or is used for *'cold sores.'* So, when a genital infection is labeled *'herpes,'* the link is made to cold sores. A condition which people find more comfortable, and less likely to alarm the patient. So, for the rest of the world, getting herpes is about as significant as getting the flu. *"We're human. We get sick. We see the doctor and most of the time we get better."*

In 2015, Duck Dynasty's Phil Robertson told the Conservative Political Action Conference (CPAC) that 110 million Americans were infected with sexually transmitted diseases and that it was *"the revenge of the hippies."* http://bit.ly/2EjxJ19. The Duck Commander continued, *"What do you call the 110 million people who have sexually transmitted illnesses? The revenge of the hippies! Sex, drugs, and rock and roll have come back to haunt us! In a bad way."*

Even without the Duck's quack-mentality, S-E-X in America is burdened with controversy, guilt, shame, and fear, despite the many hippie *"Summer-Love-Ins."* Attach herpes to sex, an 'incurable' but most often a harmless disease, and we get afraid. Unsure how the disease will impact our lives and those of loved ones. The loud silence that surrounds STDs, but mainly Genital Herpes, is not just an absence of input, but a breeding ground for isolation and shame. We cultivate the Genital Herpes stigma when we avoid talking about it openly. And like most communication blackouts, when the lights of discourse are turned on, we recognize the 'stigma' was a collective illusion. There's nothing out there except a few tweets, jokes, and myths.

The paradox: sexuality for most of us is part of our daily routine. From the clothes we wear, to the make-up women put on, the cars men drive, and movies we enjoy. It's prevalent in every venue of life. But one thing we know for certain about the Genital Herpes pharmaceutical inspired media circus: *"No one with Genital Herpes gets to be happy, unless they're on Valtrex."* Many people are uncomfortable talking about sex. That's normal given the magnitude of silence that pervades herpes and sex. Some people tend to over-correct and over-reveal in the name of honesty. And that's OK, too. But whatever you do, please don't keep silent. Go ahead, get your hippie revenge. Join the party and share. It's nothing compared to the manufactured marketing assault we're bludgeoned with every day.

B. Cold Sores (HSV-1)

Cold sores: AKA fever blisters typically appear outside the mouth, under the nose, around the lips, or underneath the chin. How bad can it be? As it turns out, **HSV-1** can be more troublesome than our HSV-2 sexual predator. Since HSV-1 involves mostly facial nerve cells, it can spread to the eyes, causing ocular herpes, which can result in blindness. In fact, ocular herpes is the most common cause of blindness in the industrial world, with over 500,000 cases reported each year in the U.S. alone. So, primp up, put in those contacts. *Sorry, not with those fingers.* Wash your hands first, thoroughly, before putting in your contacts. No matter what! Even if you don't think you have an active outbreak.

HSV-1: has also been known to infect the brain, creating a condition known as **Herpes-Simplex-Encephalitis** (HSE). It has a mortality rate of up to thirty percent (30%) with anti-vital treatment and seventy to eighty percent (70-80%) without treatment. When death happens, it's usually because of severe inflammation and brain swelling. Both conditions are a grim reminder if we're careless with HSV-1.

Historically, HSV-1 indicated oral herpes, while HSV-2 signified genital outbreaks. Due to the prevalence of oral sex the location of outbreaks is no longer a reliable indicator. In fact,

HSV-1 is increasingly found in genital cultures. **Reminder:** if you have cold sores (HSV-1), it does NOT protect you from Genital Herpes (HSV-2), why most people have both.

C. Other Oral Infections

There seems to be some confusion regarding **cold sores vs. canker sores.** Cold sores are herpes lesions. Canker sores are not. They are aphthous ulcers. Small, shallow sores found inside your mouth or at the base of the gums. As a rule, viruses and bacteria cause most oral infections. They are common, but their source and origins are difficult to diagnose. Most oral infections are not contagious, because the bacteria that usually cause them to occur naturally in our mouth. *Herpangina* is very contagious and can spread from simple contact with an infected person's mouth or nose. (See below)

Canker Sores or Aphthous Ulcers are painful but benign sores that occur on the tongue, inside the lips, cheeks, gums, and palate. There's no evidence that canker sores are caused by a virus or any infectious agent. However, they're common and often confused with mouth infections. They appear as a single or cluster of small, pale, gray-white ulcers, at times surrounded by inflamed, red tissue. Many believe that something triggers the immune system, and the cells that fight infections *"attack"* our own tissue, forming a canker sore. It's iatrogenic, meaning doctors are too *'idiotrogenic'* to figure it out, so they *'projectrogenic.'* The pain from a canker sore can last up to ten (10) days. Most heal in one to three (1 to 3) weeks. They tend to come and go throughout a person's life, unless they figure out what causes the immune response. A dermatologist or dentist can diagnose canker sores during an examination. They heal without treatment, but an array of over-the-counter products help ease their pain. Like herpes, there's no magic pill to prevent or cure canker sores.

Herpangina is an infection of painful sores on the roof of the mouth, tonsils, and/or inside the cheeks. Lesions start as small bumps, then become whitish sores with a red border. Herpangina is caused by the *coxsackie-virus*, which is also responsible for hand, foot, and mouth disease. Like most viral infections, herpangina is difficult to treat and prevent. There is no magic bullet. Some find relief by drinking plenty of water or applying an over-the-counter numbing cream. You may need the help of a qualified dermatologist to differentiate between herpes, herpangina, or aphthous ulcer/canker sores. And even though our focus is on Genital Herpes (HSV-2), the good news is that the Hermes Protocol helps all virus-related infections.

D. Genital Herpes (HSV-2)

Fluids in a herpes sore carry the virus. Contact with those fluids can spread and cause an infection. You can also get herpes from an infected sex partner who does not have a visible sore or who may not know they are infected.

Genital Herpes (HSV-2): sores usually appear as a cluster of blisters on or around the sacrum, genital/vaginal area, or buttocks (rectum). The blisters break and leave painful sores that bleed easily and often require several weeks to heal. When sores come in contact with the mouth, vagina, or rectum during sex, they can increase the risk of giving or getting HIV if either partner is infected.

Puffed-Up Stigma: For most who live with Genital Herpes it's a nonevent. For some it's a nuisance. The most challenging symptoms are *depression, isolation, and shame*. It can affect dating, social life, and psychological health. The stigma at the heart of this broken mindset is frequently worse than the symptoms. Films and TV no doubt keep Genital Herpes' social unacceptability alive. Almost every Judd Apatow movie, "*Knocked Up, Bridesmaid,* and *Trainwreck*" contains some derisive joke about herpes. But for a minority, their lives are dramatized and often exaggerated by chronic outbreaks, skin complications, and emotional complexities.

Triggers & Stages

Prodromal Stage: during the first Genital Herpes outbreak (prodromal stage), small clusters of white blisters may occur on the vagina, cervix, penis, or anus. The blisters break and leave tender sores. Symptoms include pain, fever, itching, burning, and swelling of the lymph nodes in the groin area.

Asymptomatic stage: the herpes virus lies dormant in nerve cells. At times it can reactivate and move to the surface of the skin without causing any symptoms. It's called asymptomatic viral shedding. Herpes can be transmitted even if there are no visible symptoms.

Outbreak Triggers:
1. Alcohol.
2. General illness (from mild to serious conditions).
3. Dehydration.
4. Emotional stress.
5. Fatigue.
6. Immune-compromised, from steroids, chemotherapy, or AIDS.
7. Low immunity.
8. Menstruation.

9. Poor nutrition.
10. Physical stress.
11. Sunlight, and
12. Physical trauma to the affected area.

If you've lived a life of herpes secrecy and believe that the "puffed-up stigma" is true, it's time to come out from chat-room darkness and into open-air lightness. Clear the slate and make a new beginning by declaring 'your' truth. *"I have herpes, people still like me."*

Let's stop pretending that our 'noiseless' lifestyle strategy is shyness, instead of wishing we were not infected, or hoping one day that the predator will just walk out of our life. Let's do something different today and open the curtains and windows of reality to let the sunshine in. Oops, not too much sun now. It's so exhausting to live a life of secrecy and play act that "everything is fine," when internally, we're fragile and struggling. The stress of that incongruity alone is enough to cause outbreaks. If you're unsure of how to go about taking the first step, read on. The Hermes Protocol will guide you through the process.

Yes, herpes is a natural filtering mechanism for attracting that special someone. And maybe that's not such a terrible thing. From my past experiences, the people I was attracted to were picked by my ego. Not wisdom. My ego made choices based on "feeling good" and not on what was "good for me." If we spend our time always looking to be fulfilled, versus fulfilling our purpose, it won't bode well for our happiness, or for herpetic outbreaks. When it comes to finding genuine happiness, the simplest approach is to aim your wisdom at a Higher Power. Whether we choose to call Her or Him God, or Higher Power, or Buddha, it doesn't matter as long as it's not you. No matter what faith or Higher Power we encompass, Divine Wisdom will lead the way home.

The Genital Herpes stigma is not getting better, but with COVID-19 and "now" the Monkeypox Virus taking up most of the media's attention, it's not getting worse either. Maybe over-spinning the hysteria pendulum of Genital Herpes is not such a dreadful thing. The "madness" is like a collective over-dramatized ego phenomenon. And like all ego shooting fuzzballs, they burn up when they enter the atmosphere of reality.

Convicted and Jailed

2011: David Golding, who worked for the Highways Agency in England, gave his girlfriend Genital Herpes. He was convicted and jailed for 14 months after they broke up and she reported him to the police. He initially kept quiet about his herpes STI when he began his relationship with 24-year-old Cara. Within two months she was diagnosed with HSV-2 and confronted him. Golding denied he was responsible. That was a lie.

Golding's conviction after pleading guilty to grievous bodily harm, was attacked as 'outrageous' by sexual health charities. They said the 'trivial' condition was being wrongly stigmatized. But the judge would hear none of it. *"Because herpes was transmitted in a* *relationship, it was particularly mean and an offence which amounted to a betrayal. A betrayal in a relationship in which you professed love."* Oh, my! There is a ring of truth if 'professed love' is to be open and honest.

2014: Court of Appeal rejected Golding's appeal. Lord Justice Treacy said that even though Golding had acted *"recklessly rather than deliberately"* in giving his ex the virus, his original conviction was appropriate. However, his sentence was reduced to three months. Here's an excellent example of medical professionals going head-to-head against 'Big Brother's' insatiable thirst to control every aspect of our lives and changing herpes into leprosy. Medical experts were correct in calling it out for what it really is most of the time, a trivial disease. It may be time to reconsider your stance on whether to kiss-and-tell, not-tell-and-kiss, tell-and-kiss, or not kiss at all. If discernment is difficult, the truth sets us free.

A problem with the Genital Herpes health dilemma, most pain inflicted by the herpes virus is not physical, but emotional. Having said that, please remember there is a silent minority who suffer debilitating, and at times, life threating physical symptoms that can be both emotionally draining and physically challenging.

HIV and HSV

The 2012 statistics from England show that less than 1% of those infected with HIV/AIDS died. That's about the same mortality rate as in the general population. A similar study from the US found that, *"Some groups of people with HIV now have life expectancies even higher than the US general population."* http://bit.ly/2GrkOuM

With those kinds of numbers, it's hard to argue that HIV is still an automatic death sentence. On the other hand, for many Genital Herpes sufferers, it is an emotional life sentence. Throughout HIV's brief history, Herpes & HIV have been joined at the hip. Both medicalized as a disease and moralized as a stigma. The difference is that the media hasn't turned AIDS into one-liners or comic tweets.

Social Impact: Genital Herpes is often disproportionate to its physical symptoms. Herpes patients fear more being ostracized than the virus itself. Besides rates of depression being significantly higher, recurrent Genital Herpes sufferers score higher on the Minnesota Multiphasic Personality Inventory (MMPI), suggesting not only greater depression, but anger, anxiety, worry, and interpersonal troubles.

The unfortunate part, these same stressful life events place you at higher risk for repeated herpetic episodes. And round-and-round we go, and nobody knows where and when the madness will slow. http://bit.ly/2nhQKdc

"Some of your greatest advances you have judged as failures, and some of your deepest retreats you have evaluated as success." ACIM, T-18.v.1:6

I can't think of anyone who would choose herpes as one of life's ingredients. But then we don't actively pursue divorce, cancer, or bankruptcy either. They are life's murky ingredients. When life happens, we are often shocked, confused, and plead *"Why me?"* Eventually I realized that it's *up to me* instead of *why me*. I'm responsible for what I do with my ingredients, with or without herpes or divorce. The only way out is to first accept responsibility, and the possibility that I may never heal or be married.

The secret to *"baking"* a good life with your ingredients? Don't try to discard them or push them away. They'll fester and grow, and your life will feel like a dump. Pull them closer. Acceptance is the key to transformation. The irony about pulling life closer is that resolutions and serenity are also closer.

Pharma, Doctor, & Media

Doctors often overlook the psychological toll Genital Herpes takes. They focus on treating its physical symptoms. Which is not unusual, since they spend only a few minutes with each patient. But, even when "it" does come up, herpes often gets their tongue, as they struggle with their own bias and judgments. Wordlessly perpetuating the stigma.

During the Haight-Ashbury and Woodstock (1969) days, doctors were incapable of making a distinction between HSV-1 and HSV-2. Outbreaks on your mouth or genitals were all just herpes. Then through testing, the distinction between HSV-1 and HSV-2 occurred. Instantly, the media gave birth to a "good" and "bad" virus. Herpes on the mouth indicated appropriate behavior. Genital Herpes signified immorality and sexual proclivity. After the '70s, all infectious eyes were on HIV and Herpes. HIV was considered a death sentence. Herpes an illegitimate child of the "sexual revolution." It didn't take long before the media changed a benign, but irritating virus that "itches down there," into "herpes, sexual predator." The scourge of all decent people.

1982: *Time Magazine* ran a cover story titled *"The New Scarlet Letter."* It reinforced, and armor-plated, the herpes' stigma. The authors argued that herpes would put an end to the so-called sexual revolution. *"After chastity slouched off into exile in the sixties ('60's), the sexual revolution encountered little resistance. Herpes sent thousands of sufferers spinning into months of depression and self-exile and delivered a numbing blow to the one-night stand. The herpes counter revolution may be ushering a reluctant, grudging chastity back into fashion."* http://bit.ly/2DSavBzTIME

Herpes was portrayed as a thorn in the private parts of all swingers, prostitutes, and philanderers. Women *"give husbands smiling lectures on the ravages of the disease to keep them faithful."* The piece insinuated that Genital Herpes is the righteous judgement of a moral universe and thanked herpes for *"helping to end an era of mindless promiscuity"* and *"ushering in a period in which sex is linked more firmly to commitment and trust."* Wow! Time can stand still. Let's move forward.

March 3, 2016: Haley Potiker wrote a piece on her blog entitled, *"Did Big Pharma Create the Herpes Stigma for Profit?"* http://bit.ly/2FIO1G7 Many within the *"Herpes"* community believe that Burroughs Wellcome, the company behind the drug Acyclovir (Zovirax), *"designed their advertising campaign to stimulate demand by raising patients' concerns about the social consequences and implications of infection and emphasizing that Acyclovir could reduce outbreaks and transmission. The campaign appears to have created the stigma which has clung to Genital Herpes ever since."* http://bit.ly/2DJG8OA

1983, an article in *The New York Times,* concluded, *"The current herpes epidemic presents a rare opportunity in the drug business, and thriving new market with potentially booming profits."*

E. Shingles

Shingles is another virus that can be troublesome. Related to the chickenpox virus, it behaves much like herpes, emerging in the form of blisters when the immune system is compromised. There are about one-million (1,000,000) cases of shingles each year in the U.S. alone. The risk increases for those over age fifty (50) who have a compromised immune system. Anyone who's recovered from chickenpox can get shingles, even children. It can be very painful long after the rash has disappeared. It's not contagious but can infect a person who's not had chickenpox. The good news for shingles, and there is little, the Hermes Protocols addresses and can also improve its symptoms. (Shingles Close-Up Photo Below)

F. Getting Tested

It's best to diagnose herpes at the first sign of a lesion. Get examined ASAP by a doctor if there are unusual sores, smelly discharge, a burning sensation when urinating, or bleeding for women between periods. A physician can often diagnose Genital Herpes by noting and looking at a person's symptoms. Culture is highly recommended. It will give a definitive diagnosis. Once a lesions crusts over it has poor accuracy. If the window of opportunity is missed, repeat the culture at the beginning of the next outbreak. Choose one of several options listed below. There are other skin conditions that can mimic a herpes infection: eczema, Lichen sclerosis, syphilis, molluscum contagiosum, impetigo, and yeast infections. Get evaluated to make sure it's HSV.

According to the **American Sexual Health Association** (ASHA) *"...there are different tests available for herpes. Viral culture and DNA tests can be done if you are experiencing symptoms. Blood tests are available for people who may not have symptoms or if the signs have already healed."* http://bit.ly/2DGThDD

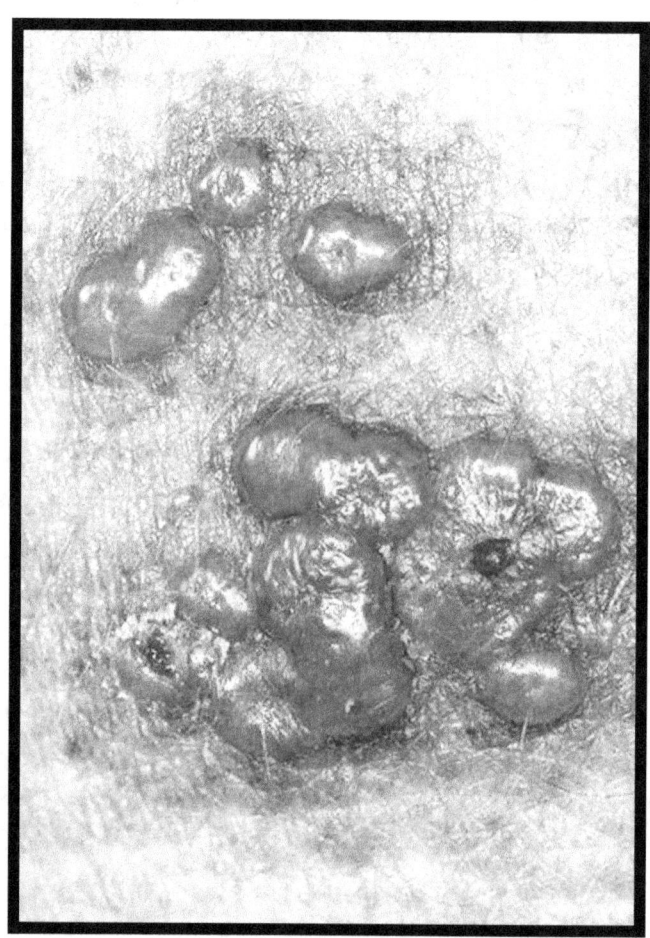

Herpes Viral Lesions Tests

If a Genital Herpes outbreak occurs, take a viral culture or a swab test within the first forty-eight (48) hours of onset. It takes about one week to get results. According to ASHA, the **herpes viral culture** test has major pros and cons. The test is known for its accuracy. If test results are positive for herpes, rest insecure. You have the virus. The test also identifies whether a person is infected with HSV-1 or HSV-2 virus. But be aware that a herpes viral culture test also has a high rate of **false negative** readings. The viral culture test needs an active virus. If the lesion has started to crust, there's a good chance of not getting an accurate reading, and of obtaining a false negative if the test is administered more than forty-eight (48) hours after symptoms appear. A viral culture of a person's *"second"* herpes outbreak is less accurate.

NAAT Test

Apart from a swab test, a Nucleic Acid Amplification Testing (NAAT) can also check for herpes. Because of speed and accuracy, and its lower risk for a false negative, NAATs are becoming the preferred method of testing. The most common NAAT method is the **Polymerase Chain Reaction or PCR** test. The test is performed on cells or fluids from a sore and/or blood or other bodily fluids. PCR tests are known for their accuracy and a 4-hour quick turnaround. The downside, they're expensive and not yet widely available.

Antibody or Blood Test

Doctors can perform an antibody or blood test to determine if a person is infected with the herpes virus even before an outbreak occurs. The test searches for immunoglobulin (IgG) antibodies in the blood. It also verifies whether it's HSV-1 or HSV-2. The antibody test is known for its accuracy. The time frame when the IgG antibodies can be detected varies from person to person. Some have detectable IgG antibody levels in weeks, others in months. There's a good chance the test will yield a false negative if a person tests too soon. ASHA advises waiting 12 to 16 weeks after exposure to ensure that antibodies can be detected. **IMPORTANT:** get evaluated before starting the Hermes Protocol.

G. Not Getting Infected

The Secret: to not getting infected with Genital Herpes is to live like David Vetter. Affectionately known as the *"boy in the bubble,"* David was born in 1971 with Severe Combined Immune Deficiency (SCID). For 12 years David captured our attention as he lived in a sterilized dome to maintain a germ-free environment. Herpes probably would have killed David. http://bit.ly/2DFWvYb Few of us are capable or willing to isolate like David Vetter just to avoid herpes. The reality is we don't have to. Most of us already have some form of the virus. Also, we can only get infected by someone who already has Genital Herpes, from one sexual encounter, whether we wear a condom or not. I repeat: condoms are little bit like locking the front door and setting the alarm. They lower the risk of getting burglarized, but it does not bullet proof getting broken into, or being infected.

Herpes sheds about ten (10) percent of the time without an outbreak, according to a recent study published in the *Journal of American Medical Association*. It matters little if the other person has symptoms or not. We can still get infected. http://bit.ly/2rQISVY With an active outbreak, try not to touch the sores or their fluids. Be especially careful around the eyes (ocular herpes) and people you come in contact with. If you accidentally touch the sores or fluids. Wash your hands! Thoroughly, to avoid spreading the infection. These cautions are repeated *ad nauseum* throughout this book.

Question? Where do you live on *"the boy in the bubble"* Vetter Curve? At what levels of isolation, restriction, protection, and justification do you exist? Yes, it's possible to avoid getting infected by the sexual predator. But it may not be worth the extreme "bubble" measures. To eliminate the herpes risk, avoid touching any other human being. Abstain from all sexual contact: vaginal, oral, anal, or other. Doesn't sound appealing or possible. But you can reduce the chance of getting infected by being in a long-term, mutually monogamous relationship. With both partners having evaluated negative. It's important to understand that *"nothing"* fully protects against herpes 100%. It occurs in both men and women's oral cavities or genital areas that are not covered by contraceptives. The mouth and tongue, or anus, rectum, perineum, and testicles.

A bit of good news for the women in our lives. A 2016 study found that contraceptive pills might be effective in fighting herpes. *"The McMaster University study in mice suggested that the female sex hormone,* **estradiol (E2),** *exerts protective effects against the herpes virus by shifting the immune response in the vaginal mucosa toward a more effective antiviral one."*

"In the past, studies have shown that injectable contraceptives containing progestins may increase a woman's risk of being infected with HIV and HSV-2. On the other hand, estradiol, another hormone that is present during the normal menstrual cycle and contained in oral contraceptives, has been shown to be protective." **CAUTION**: many people infected with herpes don't know it. They've never been evaluated, had an active outbreak, or any symptoms. Even so, they're still capable of passing it on.

H. Isolation Viral

Loneliness: is a problem for many people, but more for chronic herpes sufferers. What if we could enjoy loneliness? Change it from a negative, painful experience, to a positive one. Just as it's not the ingredients (being alone) in life, but how we relate to them that's important. So, it is with being alone. It's how our minds relate to being alone. Our herpes experience often lacks a sense of humor. I don't mean telling jokes, being funny, or criticizing other people and then laughing at them. They already do that enough to us. But having a light effect. Not beating our herpes experience into the ground. Appreciating the reality of life for what it is. Weird and wonderful, mysterious, almost humorous, and yet, it's not mocking us. With that realization we come to accept personal responsibility for uplifting our herpes experience of loneliness.

How do You Create more peace and harmony, even if infected with Genital Herpes and live alone? Loneliness doesn't destroy happiness. It's our relationship with Genital Herpes and being alone that can create feelings of loneliness if we allow it.

If we break down the barricades of shame, guilt, and feelings of isolation that envelopes herpes, then the walls of feeling lonely crumble. Herpes is now part of us. A teammate in our loneliness. It's nothing to be ashamed of. *"I have the life ingredient of herpes. I'm okay with that. People still like me, but more important, I like me."* It's how we relate to our herpes experience. We get afraid of loneliness because of our self-identification with the disease. Then it's not a stretch to think of *ourselves* as the *disease*. Very often loneliness is an identity crisis. If we're constantly identifying with our disease, even when by ourselves, we can get confused about who we are.

We all know the common stereotypes. At a certain age we're supposed to be married, have kids, lots of friends, or at least have somebody there. Being alone with any chronic disease can create an identity crisis. Feelings of failure. But herpes is special. See, we're special. Now that's something to feel good about.

The Problem with Genital Herpes is fitting it back into our life. Someone who is somebody doesn't have Genital Herpes. At least they don't admit to it. The ego-self rears its ugly head once again. Reality check! Hello. Is anybody listening? Almost everyone is infected with the herpes virus. We don't ostracize those who catch the flu. Even though its annual death toll can be as high as 48,614. Herpes is not dangerous until there is a serious health condition along with it (Eczema Herpeticum). The virus can weaken the immune system, so it can cause other health challenges.

When we get together with friends, kindred spirits, we have an identity. The lonely self is somebody in a crowd of supporters. Then we get into our cars and drive home alone. Sorry, we've just left our identity behind. Triggering a strange, barren feeling of loneliness. There's no freedom relying on happiness from the ever shifting and changing **outside world**. It's an identity crisis when we define ourselves by our relationships, marriage, family, job, and physical appearance. But even worse, if by our disease, Genital Herpes.

Why is there so much pain and grief in divorce? Because we not only lose a loved one but also our identity of being a supportive wife or husband. The world around us encourages us to make identities. I am a plumber, a firefighter, husband, she's my wife, and who are you? I'm a Genital Herpes carrier. Bummer. No wonder you feel alone. What a world. Thank you for manufacturing our identity. Better yet, I'll go out and buy some drugs or take an antidepressant.

It starts early in grammar school. He's the clown, or he's the smart one, she's the pretty one, and soon we *"identify with their identity."* From then on, every day, in every way, we are bombarded by the media to *"fix"* our identity. You don't have to be any of those things. Experiment letting go of all your identification. Being a woman or man, rich or poor, young, or old, a Democrat or Republican, sick, or healthy. Even though the body is sick with herpes, the mind doesn't have to be. And if the checkbook is empty, the mind can be full of compassion. Try it for a week. See what it feels like.

A good place to start is with **Chapter 12: Psychology of Health.** We don't need to identify with our disease. It's mind-blowing to see an extremely sick person laughing, telling jokes, being at peace. But it can be done. It has been done by many throughout history. Here are a couple of extreme examples.

During the persecution of the Christians, St. Lawrence was condemned to a slow, cruel death. The Saint was tied to an iron grill over a slow fire that roasted his flesh little by little. History tells us he almost did not feel the flames. In fact, it's said he joked, telling the judge, *"Turn me over, I'm done on this side!"* And just before he died, *"It's cooked enough now."* Then he prayed that Rome might be converted, and that the Faith spread all over the world. Saint Lawrence's feast day is August 10th.

June 11, 1963: Vietnamese Buddhist monk Thích Quang Duc immolated himself at a busy Saigon road intersection to protest the war, setting himself on fire and burning to death without so much as a whimper. Surely, if he can do that we can transcend loneliness. How can you be lonely if you are your best friend? **A**re you? Maybe you're an adversary. It's something to consider when we look at why we feel lonely.

When we're alone, can we stop running away from ourselves? Face who we are. Let go of the self-business, the me! The *I'm a this and I'm a that*. I'm sick with Genital Herpes. Let all that manure go. Compost your garden instead. Realize the body has herpes, you do not. Yes, the body might be unattractive, but you're not. The body might be old, but not you. We can't control the body with its ailments, just as we can't control the ingredients of life.

Spiritual Power: not the false sense of control power, is the way to peace and happiness. It's in our relationship to People, Places, and Things wherein lies the problem and solution.

Chapter 4: Eczema Herpeticum

Before 2015, Genital Herpes was just inconvenient, emotionally draining. That changed with my first eczema flare-up. I had no idea how troublesome eczema can be for those infected with the herpes virus. With eczema there are potential triggers that make symptoms worse. What is relatively unknown is the most dangerous trigger is herpes. Either cold sores or Genital Herpes. Who knew? My general practitioner (GP) never said a word. Most GPs are unfamiliar with the complications of having eczema and herpes break out at the same time. They don't see it enough. It's more in the realm of textbook dermatology or infectious disease. Please be vigilant if you're infected with both herpes and eczema. Eczema Herpeticum can be a mess, waiting for a train wreck.

Eczema Herpeticum (EH): develops when eczema-damaged skin is infected with HSV-1 or HSV-2. A herpes infection on an eczematous area of the skin can quickly spread into a painful, blistery, oozing rash. An out-of-control brush fire. If left untreated, it can spread to vital organs throughout the body. On rare occasions it is still fatal. October 2016 when Genital Herpes and eczema turned ugly for the author. *(Photograph below. Author's Infection with Eczema Herpeticum, November 2016)*

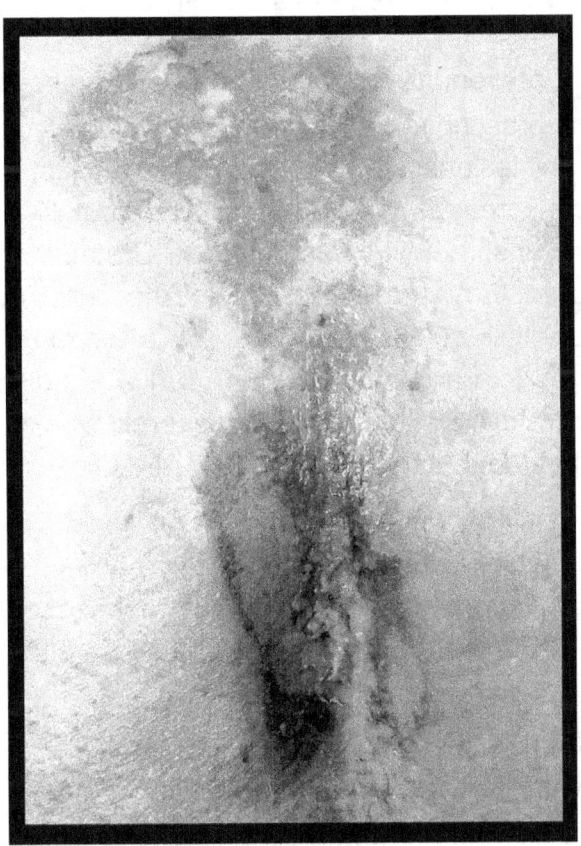

Most often herpes and eczema are two separate diseases. Bothersome, but they seldom cause serious complications. Most herpes outbreaks and eczema flare-ups heal on their own without difficulties. With one grave exception: when an eczema flare-up, usually atopic dermatitis (AD), is infected with the herpes virus (HSV-1 or HSV-2). A chance encounter can develop into Eczema Herpeticum. A rare, but serious, and even fatal infection if treatment is not properly initiated.

Technically, *Herpeticum* is a form of Kaposi Varicelliform Eruption (KVE). A blistery rash that usually arises from atopic dermatitis (AD). Eczema Herpeticum can be severe, progressing from a single rash/outbreak into an infection that quickly spreads throughout the body. http://bit.ly/2DJl35r It's important to be diagnosed early and treated promptly. The most common treatment is antiviral medication that varies in dose depending on the patient's immune status. To diagnose Eczema Herpeticum (EH) doctors swab the lesions and culture it.

"Just like other HSV infections, Eczema Herpeticum can recur. In immune compromised patients the mortality rate is reported to be as high as 6% to 10% and even 50%. Timely diagnosis and treatment of Eczema Herpeticum is important to avoid severe complications." http://bit.ly/2DJXdnl Since Eczema Herpeticum is uncommon, it's sometimes misdiagnosed as impetigo. A detailed history can make a difference for an accurate diagnosis. Even though other viruses cause herpeticum, it's most frequent with herpes infections. That's why it's referred to as Eczema Herpeticum (EH).

EH can require long-term preventative treatment. My outbreaks lasted from October 2016 to April 2017. My doctor prescribed Acyclovir and a topical anti-bacterial cream, to be applied as necessary to any lesions. At first, I thought it was just a severe case of eczema. But as the rash and ulcers spread, my sacrum started to look like the endgame of a World War II flame thrower. I knew something was different. Gratefully, so did my doctors. Even though nothing was cultured, they were pre-emptive. After applying the ointment, I covered the lesions with large non-stick sterile Band-Aids. EH's rash surrounded my sacrum and anus. Number *"two"* turned into a two-hour clean up. I was not hospitalized because I'm stubborn but took oral antiviral therapy for several weeks. Advanced cases are hospitalized and put on intravenous treatment.

It's been eight months since my last herpes or EH outbreak. The doctors warned me that long-term outcomes are inconsistent and recurrence rates high. I was to remain vigilant and prepared for regular therapy. Lesions and outbreaks healed slowly, and at times worsened until I started the Hermes Protocol (see Chapters 10 to 13).

Although EH occurred on my sacrum with HSV-2, it's more often caused by cold sores (HSV-1) with eczema flare-ups on the face, neck, or upper trunk. Symptoms of EH do not appear right away. They typically show up a week or two after being infected with the herpes virus. Eczema Herpeticum symptoms can include a blistery rash that appears in clusters and often covers a large area. The blister can break open, be itchy, painful, weep, bleed, and/or have pus-like yellow fluid inside. As the rash appears, it feels like the flu with swollen lymph nodes, fever, chills, and fatigue.

Complications may involve:

1. Long-term scarring from slow healing blisters.

2. A herpes infection in the cornea of the eye, known as herpetic keratitis, can lead to blindness if left untreated.

3. Let me stress, prompt treatment is essential. If herpes spreads to your brain, lungs, or liver, organ failure may occur. I'm not sure we want to live without our brain, liver, or even our lungs. Well, at times I wouldn't mind living without my critical brain.

Herpeticum frequently occurs with these skin conditions:

1. Atopic Dermatitis (AD)
2. Seborrheic Dermatitis
3. Irritant Contact Dermatitis
4. Burns
5. Psoriasis

EH's primary victims are infants and children. However, anyone with a compromised immune system is fair game and susceptible. With eczema, please avoid contact with anyone who has a cold sore or Genital Herpes. Those with partners may want to sleep in the guest room or couch. Wait until the abscess leaves the heart fonder. Do not share eating utensils, cosmetics, clothing, glassware, or any other item that touched active herpes lesions.

"What to do if in a relationship?"

1. Keep herpes infections under control.
2. Keep eczema flare-ups under control.
3. If you're both active, avoid contact with others

Suggestions that may help:

Know your triggers. It may be easier to avoid eczema flare-ups than herpes outbreaks. Or it may not. Avoid both whenever possible. With an active eczema flare-up, ask your doctor whether it's a good idea to take antiviral meds until the eczema subsides. It may keep herpes from breaking out at the same time, in the same spot.

Avoid scratching your skin. It may cause cracks or breaks, leaving it vulnerable to infections. Coconut oil is both a moisturizer and protectant.

Use herpes and/or eczema medications as prescribed. Both oral and topical creams can promote eczema healing, relieve itching and inflammation. With an active Genital Herpes outbreak, be careful. Creams beneficial to eczema may not be for herpes. Eczema corticosteroid creams come in different strengths, from mild *over the counter* (OTC) treatments, to strong prescription medicines. For Genital Herpes, I used an MMS and DMSO solution several times a day to resolve symptoms (Chapter 10, MMS and DMSO). Keep track of your herpes and eczema symptoms. *Always* see a doctor if they worsen! Especially if a fever is present.

Protect affected skin with a non-stick Band-Aid, especially near the sacrum. Wash hands frequently and avoid direct contact with lesions whenever possible. Use a Q-Tip for medication ointments or creams. Avoid sex with an active outbreak. No matter what, make sure to wear protection. A latex condom acts as a barrier against sexually transmitted infections, including herpes. But like anything else in life, except death and time, it's not a guarantee. Although our focus is Genital Herpes, the Hermes Protocol helped both herpes and eczema: **Eczema Herpeticum.** 2016, Reinhard Hermes, Low Back Eczema Herpeticum Outbreak.

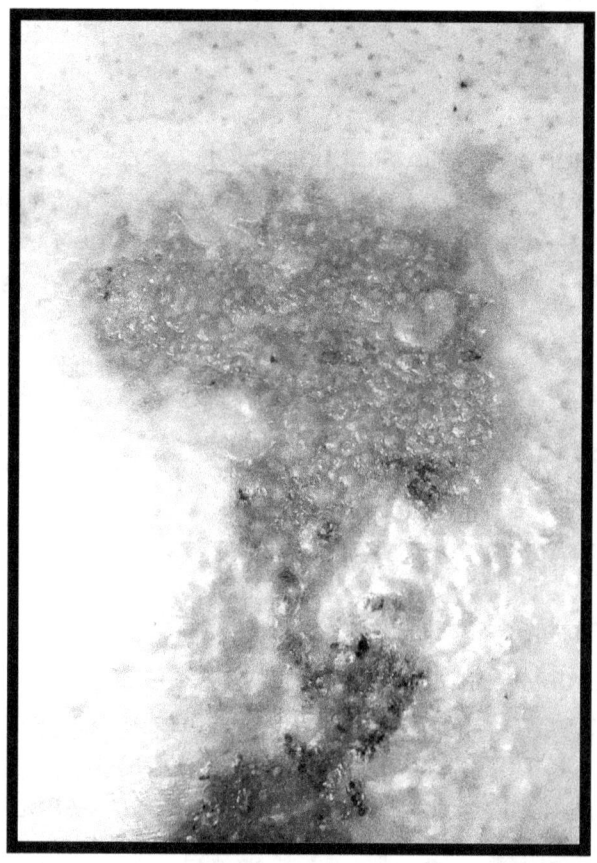

2016 Herpes & Eczema = Eczema Herpeticum

Chapter 5: Orthodox Medicine

1980s 'Cheers' reruns are entertaining, but I get woozy watching the re-runs of *'happy Valtrex days are here again'* infomercials. A handsome young couple skipping hand-in-hand through an idyllic field of California wildflowers. Eyeing the camera, they're barely able to contain their lustful gleam. Like two giggling cannabis euphoric teens, they're seen loping into the horizon to have the best Valtrex sex of their lives. *Oops, sorry,* almost forgot. Both actors have active lesions. And even Valtrex can't erase that pain. Unless, of course, they also have a script for Oxycodone. The paradox, we remember the thirty percent (30%) *"live happily ever after parts,"* not the medical jargon, disclosing a litany of nasty side effects.

The biggest deceptions in drug advertising are not falsified scientific studies or out-and-out lies. It's their distorted realities and visual allusions that assail us daily. Underplaying drug's serious risks. Like any propaganda, if ads are repeated enough we eventually disconnect, tune out warnings, or focus only on what 'they want us to see.' The happy couple, and *"litany of disclaimer side-effects can't be that bad, not if you should 'ask your doctor'."* Incidentally, unlike drug advertisements, the FDA does not regulate *"disease awareness"* promotions. For example, cheesy TV soap opera scripts are often deceptive drug ads. A leading character comes down with a life-threatening viral infection and sees their health restored by a drug company, who happens to have an Rx antiviral for that.

The FDA: guardians of our health and well-being. Watch dog of our food supply. A marionette for the puppet masters: Pig Pharma, Pig Agri, Pig Government, and BIG money. It's incestuous. Play the *"game"* well enough and get promoted. Then elected to office, and eventually work for the FDA. We underwrite their *"duplicity"* with our vote, tax dollars, and the drugs and food we purchase. What an Oscar performance. Nowhere else are their concerts sold out. But everyone denies playing their part. It reminds me of Lewis Carroll's poem, *"The Jabberwocky,"* in *Alice in Wonderland.* It's all gibberish to me. And the lines between illegal and legal are more blurred than ever now that *legal* prescription drugs kill more than all illegal street drugs combined. So, when did medicine's Hippocratic Oath change to the Hypocrites Oath. From *"First do no harm"* to *"First make money?"* When did American lives become cheaper than those of everywhere else?

Questions raised by Ron Unz, publisher of *The American Conservative.* He did a piece comparing how China dealt with their melamine baby formula drug scandal, to how the U.S. managed the Vioxx cover-up disaster. http://bit.ly/2DNAYAM *"The Chinese scandal surfaced in 2008, shortly before the Beijing Olympics. Crooked dairy farmers* diluted their milk products, and then added a plastic chemical compound called melamine to raise the apparent protein content back to normal levels. Nearly 300,000 babies across China suffered urinary problems, with many hundreds requiring lengthy hospitalization for kidney stones. Six died."

"**Long prison sentences** were handed down. Some were tried and executed. Throughout these events, American media coverage was extensive. Sneering about the Chinese leadership's indifference to human life." Four years earlier, in September 2004, Merck suddenly issued a recall for Vioxx, a pain medication to treat arthritis-related ailments. The recall came a few days before the FDA was going to release a study that indicated Vioxx significantly increased the risk of fatal strokes and heart attacks. It's estimated that over a five-year period more than 60,000 American lost their lives. Some say the range was closer to 500,000 deaths.

The sinister part was verified in the many ensuing lawsuits; that Merck knew all along of the many lethal side effects *before* it introduced Vioxx in 1999. The reason Vioxx was not pulled sooner? It became Merck's bestseller. Generating over two billion dollars ($2,000,000,000) in yearly revenue. Twenty-five million (25,000,000) Americans were prescribed Vioxx as an aspirin-substitute, under the false marketing (manufactured) belief that it produced fewer side effects. Considering the magnitude of the scandal and the number of people who lost their lives, why was it a *non-media-event?* Merck news stories were lost in the back pages with advertising. Accidental? Pharma money at work protecting specialness?

The class-action lawsuit dragged its way through the courts and was eventually **settled** in **2007** for **$4.85 billion.** What did Merck learn? Unlike the guilty parties in China, some who lost their lives, Merck's poor, misunderstood CEO was forced to resign. But he kept every penny of his $50 million compensation and was promptly replaced by one of his top lieutenants. Neither he nor any Merck crony was ever charged with a crime. When did the Hippocratic Oath become hypocritical and Chinese lives more valuable?

A. First Outbreak

"You have no future in the past." – RH

Only irresponsible, promiscuous, dirty *"hippie"* types get infected with Genital Herpes. Yes, that's true. Why wouldn't they? There's one slight problem. Even responsible, faithful, *"Mother-Theresa types"* get infected. A consistently false and exaggerated 'media' judgement is that a person must sleep with a legion of *"undesirables"* or *"hippie"* types to get infected. Truth be, it doesn't take an orgy of sexual gluttony. Only one itsy-bitsy act, with one infected, spiritual partner, to be exposed to the herpes virus.

Herpes can gain entrance to our body by touching, kissing, or vaginal, anal, and oral sex. Any break in the skin admits entry. Wash your hands. Especially with an active outbreak. In this way we don't spread the virus to other parts of the body or anyone else. Before pointing out or accusing your current partner; remember, it's conceivable to have been infected with HSV-2 for many months or even years, before suffering your first outbreak.

Most Genital Herpes outbreaks occur below the waist: on the sacrum, vulva, penis, or rectum. My lesions started on my penis. Afterwards ninety percent (90%) of the outbreaks occurred on the sacrum. Like a fingerprint, a person's response to the disease is physically and emotionally unique. Yet, underneath our differences, we have a common history. A compromised immune system. The Hermes Protocol addresses both the cause and its unique symptoms. If part of our emotional response is feeling impure, contaminated, and irresponsible, even though we know that we did nothing wrong. It may be time to push the herpes mental health reset button of forgiveness.

If you're still struggling with *"The Enemy,"* please get over being infected. Otherwise, herpes will be a minor nuisance compared to what the mind will drag you through. Save yourself a lot of mental anguish and embrace the Psychology of Health in Chapter 12.

It's important to *"get over it,"* but do not sweep herpes under the rug and pretend it never happened. With the next outbreak, look at the blisters and think of them as nothing more than another "shovel of dirt." Remember, you're not a virus. You're an ol' mule. Let's recap the most common Genital Herpes *"first-outbreak"* flu-like symptoms (HSV-1 or HSV-2) and see which apply to your history:

1. Fever
2. Chills
3. Exhaustion
4. Nerve pain
5. Body aches
6. Swollen glands

Immune compromised individuals, who suffer from complicated and/or multiple herpes infections, can have these outbreak symptoms in the first year. However, their intensity and duration tend to decrease over time and become less pronounced. Although everyone's symptoms are unique, they tend to be worse for females, including experiencing more Urinary Tract Infections (UTI). The first days of a Genital Herpes infection can be unpleasant and take two or three weeks to heal. *Please!* See your primary care physician ASAP and get evaluated and treated if necessary. It can take three (3) months to show up in bloodwork, and why a culture at the first sign is ASAP preferred.

I'm not a doctor. This book is my experience and not a substitute for seeing one. Acyclovir is recognized as the first line of defense and treatment of choice for Genital Herpes. Don't resist taking it, especially if there is pain or difficulty urinating. Antiviral prescriptions can be expensive and may not be covered by insurance. Make sure your doctor or pharmacist knows generic brand options. Wal-Mart pharmacies are a cost-effective choice. If uninsured, **Planned Parenthood** is an alternative. For more information contact Planned Parenthood at **(800) 230-7526.**

Traditional Pharmaceutical Antivirals can be taken daily and make it less likely (but not guaranteed) to pass the infection to your sex partner(s). Mainstream medicine's standard of care is antivirals, such as Acyclovir or Valtrex. They have been known to:

1. Eliminate outbreaks entirely.
2. Diminish them to a rare occurrence, and
3. Alleviate suffering significantly.

Their downside: certain individuals carry a great deal of risk for serious complications. Taking them depends on your risk-reward threshold. They did not work well for me because of their side effects. According to allopathic or mainstream medicine, there is no cure for herpes; the only option is to take suppressive retroviral pharmaceutical drugs indefinitely. See Risks and Side Effects in section D below.

Herpes is our coal mine canary. A native brook trout for a stream. Both are warning signs of potential dangers in their habitat. The *"turkey thermometer"* for the body's immune system. When the immune system is compromised and health failing, the viral hunter takes aim, and bulls' eye! The sexual predator has broken out, and no matter how hard we try to keep it locked up, it keeps breaking out. If only Pandora hadn't pilfered that key.

To give our body a fighting chance against a formidable foe, start with lifestyle choices. Yes, there's that dirty word again. *Lifestyle.* A long-winded acronym for *"No fun, no way!"* For many it's the most difficult part of the Hermes Protocol. Like asking an alcoholic to join us for *Perrier* at Happy Hour. Or a one-armed, Facebook, iPhone tweeting junky to handwrite a letter. I've heard it said it's easier to change a person's religion than their lifestyle. It depends on how much suffering we can take.

When herpes infections occur, start looking for some connections between stress, food allergies, alcohol, sun exposure, medications, constipation, or any other variable that activates outbreaks. Topicals help, but they're like pulling out the smoke alarm to douse a fire. It may drown out the noise, but it won't do much to extinguish the flames. Herpes is the fire alarm, a blinking red light in the immune system's dashboard. It's warning us to slow down, change our ways, or stop. *"Danger, Will Robinson, danger."* Life is too stressful, and the body has been pushed beyond its immune limits.

A 'Positive' Exception: to a sudden increase in outbreaks can also be a *"healing crisis."* For example, starting an antiviral like Valtrex, the body has more ammunition to put Genital Herpes back in Pandora's box. Herpes fights back, increases its viral shedding, and more outbreaks occur. A healing crisis is beneficial, and not a regression of well-being. The difficult part is differentiating between crisis or regression occurrence.

Dr. Max Gerson's Cancer workshop in San Diego, CA, emphasized treating the *"whole person"* and not just the cancer, or symptoms. According to Max Gerson, MD, a German physician, disease occurs in the body because of *"toxicity and deficiency."* A healing crisis is a common occurrence when the body starts to absorb essential nutrients and begins to eliminate toxins.

If you're anything like me, you've already spent and exceeded the national debt limit looking for Ty Bollinger's next **"Quest for the Herpes Cure."** Ty, if you're reading this, here's an idea for your next six-day infomercial. For years, I scoured the internet, trying one magic potion and remedy after another. The only thing I ever uncovered was an empty checkbook, fading hope, and more outbreaks. I've tried most pills, salves, tonics, supplements, *"cures"* and frauds, hoping to heal what modern medicine says is incurable. I never gave up. Today, in 2023 I've been outbreak free for six (6) years.

However, my healing journey did not go from *"poor me"* to *"whoopee,"* or worthlessness to self-worth. Instead, it was a resolve that turned into a *"drive"* to support a compromised immune system and turn it into a juggernaut. As you know, surface or superficial solutions seldom stopped the predator from its game. Only when I delved deeper and supported my immune system did I go into remission. Before jumping into mainstream medicine, let me reiterate mine. *"You have no future in the past."* **None.** If you find yourself besides yourself, angry and resentful that *'somebody done you wrong.'* It's time to bury the hatchets and get on with your life.

B. Antiviral Medications

Acyclovir: (Siting, Zovirax):

The oldest of four antiviral drugs. It inhibits herpes by disrupting its DNA replication and comes in a variety of application methods, including pill form and ointment. I was prescribed Acyclovir for Genital Herpes with these instructions:

1. **Initial Acyclovir treatment** for Genital Herpes was 200 mg every four hours while awake (five times daily) for ten days, or 400 mg every eight hours for seven-to-ten days.

2. **Intermittent treatment for recurrences** was 200 mg by mouth every four hours while awake (five times daily) for five days. Started at the earliest sign of symptoms.

3. Chronic suppression for recurrence was 400 mg by mouth every twelve hours for one-year, or 200 mg three-to-five times daily. I was NOT able to continue suppressive therapy because of acute side effects. I ended up in the ER on too many occasions with skyrocketing blood pressure.

Valtrex (ValAcyclovir):

Valtrex common side effects include headaches, nausea, stomach pain, vomiting, and dizziness. The antiviral commercial with happy looking couples a bit too cheerful about their diagnoses.

Famvir (Famciclovir):

Famvir is an antiviral that can slow the spread of herpes symptoms. It's especially useful for herpes zoster (shingles), strong herpes outbreaks, and a suppressed immune system because of HIV. It seems less toxic based on the potency of its side effects.

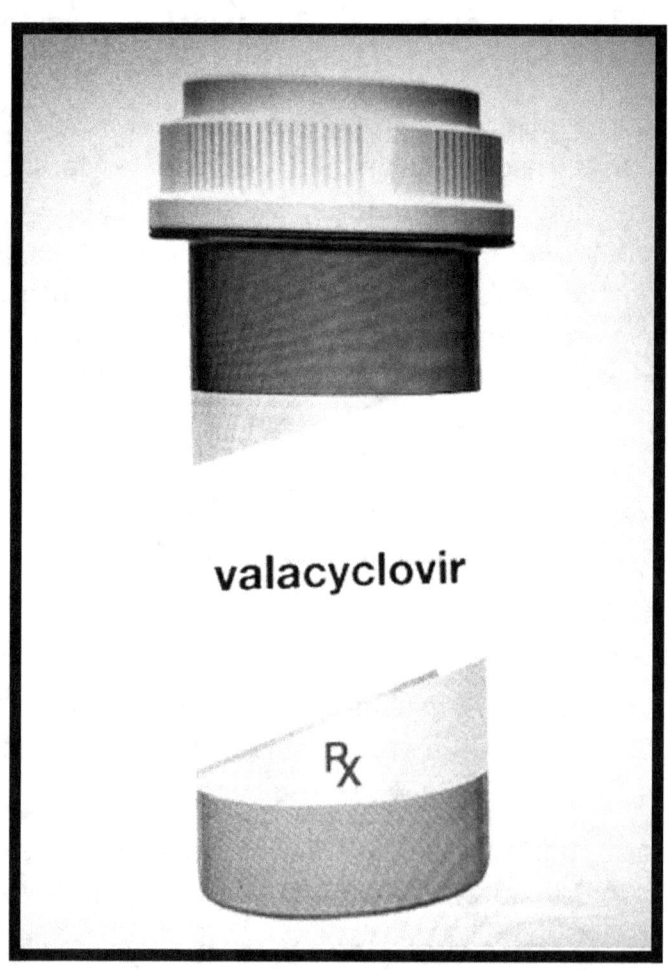

C. Every Day or As Needed

"Every Day or As Needed" is not like deciding what socks to wear with what shoes. I don't think twice about taking a daily multi-vitamin. Taking daily *"suppressive"* antiviral therapy rings different today. But only because I experienced terrible side effects. But I'm tainted by my history. I stopped suppressive antiviral therapy because I got tired of going to the Emergency Room. All medications have some inherent safety risks. Although antivirals are generally well tolerated, the internet is littered with unfortunate souls who found out too late to be cautious when taking any medication. No matter what your doctor or anyone else tells you, stay alert and cautious. Be extremely careful if you have any kidney or liver issues.

Some refuse medications on divine principles, while for others, the cost is often too prohibitive. A few *killjoys*, who are constantly on the go, find daily dosing inconvenient; however, many choose daily antiviral suppressive therapy. Even if they must put up with minor side effects because it gives them less stress, anxiety, and more peace of mind.

I was hoping to be one of the lucky ones. I was not. In retrospect, today I am the lucky one. Yet many rely on suppressive therapy, not thinking twice about "popping" their Valtrex like a multi-vitamin. There are no long-term safety studies about its side effects. The longest study I found was for one year. Something to consider before jumping in with both lesions. http://bit.ly/2Gq45rO

The University of Maryland had an excellent article about *"Nutrition and Dietary Supplements for Herpes,"* which examined several alternative treatment options. http://bit.ly/2ni1gkC However, if you clicked on the link after March 2022 you received a message of *"Page Is No Longer Available, or Internal Error."* I wonder what made them remove the Alternative Medicine content. I can only guess.

Whether to initiate suppressive treatment is often influenced by the frequency of outbreaks, severity of symptoms, and the risk of infecting an uninfected partner. The good news about the unwelcome news: over time outbreaks normally decrease, and symptoms become less severe.

D. Risks & Side Effects

All medications have risks. Most who take antiviral medication have few side effects, or minor ones. The most common are:

1. Feeling sick and nauseous.
2. Vomiting.
3. Diarrhea and/or abdominal pain.
4. Breaking out in skin rashes.
5. Including photosensitivity, and
6. Itching.

Some have serious reactions. Then there are those with liver or kidney disease, who probably should not take antivirals unless it's an absolute life or death situation. Inadequate hydration also increases the chances of kidney failure. Drink plenty of water to stay well hydrated when taking antivirals. Early warning signs of kidney problems decreased urination and kidney flank pain. Kidney pain often feels like lower back pain. Other symptoms include loss of appetite, difficulty thinking clearly, dizziness, headaches, metallic taste in your mouth, fatigue, and itchiness.

Valtrex (approved 1995) and Acyclovir (1982) can cause liver damage in some patients. Signs of liver inflammation include yellowing of the skin and eyes. The elderly, and those with a compromised immune system, may not tolerate Valtrex. Please tell your doctor if you have kidney or liver problems before taking any medication.

Technical Abstracts and Studies:

1. **Acyclovir Studies** http://bit.ly/2rHWIZk
2. **Valtrex Studies** http://bit.ly/2BAnVNl
3. **Herpes Simplex Virus** http://bit.ly/2niNQEY

Existing antiviral medications do not *"successfully"* inhibit viral replication. With suppressive therapy they reduce transmission of the herpes virus by only 50%, and at times are not adequate for more severe, potentially fatal cases, such as encephalitis and neonatal herpes.

Valtrex is often prescribed for long-term (months to years) suppression of HSV outbreaks. Valtrex has been involved with over 10,000 patients in clinical trials of up to one-year in duration. There is confidence in its long-term safety at doses up to one-thousand milligrams a day (1000 mg/day).

Acyclovir, on the other hand, has been evaluated for ten-years in a wide range of patients with recurrent Genital Herpes infections. To date, resistance to Acyclovir is rare. The effectiveness and safety of Acyclovir and Valtrex are maintained long term, or acute treatment for many years.

Famciclovir (Famvir, approved 1997) is the newest member of the three *medications*. From observational and anecdotal reports, Famvir is well tolerated. Currently, there are no known *"severe"* side effects. However, it should be noted there are also no long-term studies. Therefore, its side effects may not be fully known. The most serious Famvir risk is an allergic reaction:

1. Wheezing.
2. Difficulty Breathing.
3. Hives.
4. Swelling in the lips, throat, tongue, and
5. Muscle Pain.

Those with impaired kidney or liver function should be cautious and consider taking a lower dose. Patients with liver damage are advised against taking Famvir, or to be extremely cautious.

E. Strategies on the Horizon

According to the September 2016 issue of *Pharmaceutical Journal*, current treatments of genital or oral herpes is limited to antiviral medications, *"Which are only 50% effective at reducing transmission. New treatments are desperately needed."* Here are four of the most promising strategies on the horizon. http://bit.ly/2DI5YhP

Helicase Primase Inhibitors (HPI)

HPI is a new class of antivirals that are more advanced in inhibiting viral replication. Their purpose is to treat severe cases of Genital Herpes. Because of safety concerns their use for routine Genital Herpes dosing is still under consideration. One HPI by a Japanese company is in phase III trials, but no results have been released.

Preventative vaccines

Vaccines have protected millions from many infectious diseases, but not herpes. Despite fifty (50) years of trying, a preventative vaccine has eluded scientists. However, a new vaccine candidate has emerged.

Anna Wald, a herpes specialist from the University of Washington, says the data is "very exciting." A research team from the Albert Einstein College of Medicine in New York demonstrated in mice that the experimental new vaccine provided complete protection against a variety of HSV-1 and HSV-2 strains. http://bit.ly/2DI5YhP **Wald** cautioned that it's *"very hard to tell if a vaccine will work in humans from animals; it's easier to prevent infection in a mouse."* If all goes well, researchers hope to begin small clinical trials.

CRISPR/Cas9

CRISPR/Cas9 is a gene-editing tool that targets and cuts out specific sections of DNA. Researchers are using the technique to target the herpes virus and cripple its ability to replicate. The idea is to "eliminate the virus completely." The strategy has had some success treating HIV in pre-clinical studies. Researchers have adapted the technology to target herpes and are currently studying it in animal models. Although results are not yet available, they said it's looking *"very promising."* If all goes well, treatment will be available for patients in less than five years. It could be used for whoever has the herpes virus.

Free Clinical Trials

FREE experimental antiviral drugs unless you're taking a placebo. There are several new treatments on the horizon, but it may be years before they are available. The process of introducing a new drug is long and not without trial and error. Rigorous clinical trials are divided into three phases:

1. **Phase I,** the safety phase to determine if the drug is nontoxic.
2. **Phase II,** researchers try to find out if the drug works as it should.
3. **Phase III,** research to include more patients in more places.

To conduct trials, scientists need volunteers. Often thousands. The FDA and an independent review board carefully monitor every aspect of a trial so it's not another Vioxx disaster. Volunteers have clearly defined rights and the right to drop out at any time. If interested, the National Institutes of Health has an online database. Their website provides detailed information on how to get involved in a clinical trial.

https://www.clinicaltrials.gov/

F. Leaky Gut

People are surprised to learn that many of their mysterious and chronic health issues are often related to **intestinal permeability**, or *"leaky gut."* The old Hippocrates saying that *"All disease begins in the Gut,"* is being confirmed repeatedly by ongoing research. In a *"gutshell,"* that beer-belly is your immune system. Although diet is the number one reason for a leaky gut, high blood sugar, chronic stress, and hormonal imbalances contribute. Innocent over-the-counter remedies, such as aspirin, ibuprofen, and naproxen can wreak havoc on the stomach and intestinal lining.

Leaky Gut: is a condition in which the walls of the small intestine become inflamed, damaged, and porous. It then allows undigested foods, medicines, bacteria, yeast, and other pathogens to enter the bloodstream. When the gates from the intestines to the bloodstream "leak," foreign particles enter the bloodstream that shouldn't be there. Leaky gut is associated with food sensitivities, Inflammatory Bowel Disease (IBD), nutritional deficiencies, skin conditions, chronic disease, allergies, autoimmunity, mood disorders, autism, and more, and more, and more. Common symptoms include joint pain, gut problems, fatigue, depression, and other brain-related disorders.

What Causes Leaky Gut?

1. NSAIDs (non-steroidal anti-inflammatory drugs),
2. Opioids,
3. Antibiotics,
4. Antiviral medications,
5. Birth control pills,
6. Food toxins from grains and legumes,
7. Excess carbohydrate and fructose consumption,
8. Excess polyunsaturated and omega-6 fat consumption,
9. Infections (h-Pylori, Candida),
10. Chronic stress,
11. Lack of sleep,
12. Nutritional deficiencies, critical vitamins, minerals, and ,
13. A weak immune system (often caused by all the above).

The Question: *"What came first: Valtrex or the leaky gut?"* Did the antiviral cause the leaky gut, which triggered an allergic reaction, or was it the frequent use of antibiotics? In health-related issues, association does not necessarily mean cause. For example, after taking Acyclovir for a Genital Herpes outbreak, my blood pressure suddenly skyrocketed like the space shuttle. The doctor in the emergency room declared it an allergic reaction to Acyclovir. While that association may be true, the cause was the antibiotics from last week's dental work, which triggered the leaky gut that allowed the Acyclovir to enter the blood stream, which in turn elevated the blood pressure. The cause was leaky gut. The association, Acyclovir.

June 12, 2017: an article at **www.medscape.com** asserted that *Antibiotic-Associated-Adverse-Events* **(ADEs)** are common. One in five patients hospitalized at John Hopkins Hospital from September 2013 to June 2014 experienced an adverse event (ADEs) within the first 30 days after receiving *antibiotics*. These included:

1. Gastrointestinal
2. Dermatologic
3. Musculoskeletal
4. Hematologic
5. Hepatobiliary (Liver)
6. Renal (Kidneys)
7. Cardiac
8. Neurological Events

In addition, researchers found that one-out-of-five who received antibiotics shouldn't have. The take-home message: *"Danger, Will Robinson, danger!"* Be very, very careful when weighing the decision whether to take antibiotics. They are dangerous and *"lend further credence to the importance of antibiotic stewardship to optimize patient safety."* JAMA, Intern Med. Published online June 12, 2017. Once permeable, a leaky gut can be repaired by eating a proper diet that stabilizes blood sugar, reducing physical and mental stress, and eliminating medications that degrade leaky gut further.

Chapter 6: White-Coat Hunters

Herpes is a nonevent compared to the suffering and fatalities inflicted by modern medicine and the *Great White-Coat Hunters*. A phrase that once emphasized the racial and colonial aspects of the profession but now echoes the privileged status of the man in a *"White-Coat"* and stethoscope instead of a rifle. But the results remain the same. A lot of grieving. It's exaggerated, because the microscope of concern should focus on the influence of pharmaceutical companies, not doctors. But then again, how many drug ads end with, *"Ask your doctor versus pharmaceutical representative."*

Herpes is a virus, not a ratings barometer or Disneyland "E" ticket to sell more drugs to a duped public. Yes, there are occasions when it's prudent to take pharmaceutical drugs, but when three out five Americans are on some sort of Rx prescription, it's time to question the reason. Or better yet, the motive. Conventional medicine kills more people *"accidently-on-purpose"* than cancer, heart disease, drunk drivers, illicit drugs, etc. etc. combined.

Nutrition Institute of America professors Gary Null and Dorothy Smith, along with doctors Carolyn Dean, Martin Feldman and Debora Rosio titled their report *"Death by Medicine."* The documentary was available on YouTube http://bit.ly/2FqEg9v, (but no longer). *"The researchers found that America's leading cause of death isn't heart disease or cancer. Its conventional medicine. The iatrogenic death rate in the US (death caused by doctors and/or medical treatments) is 783,936 a year."* Download the PDF http://bit.ly/2BzrnrC.

The next ten years iatrogenic deaths will kill *"more than all the casualties from all the wars fought by the US throughout its entire history."* A death rate equivalent to six jumbo jets falling out of the sky every day. Many believe the numbers are much higher because only five-to-twenty percent (5% to 20%) of iatrogenic deaths are reported for fear of lawsuits. Codes for reporting deaths due to drugs and medical errors in many cases don't exist. The actual figures may be twenty (20) times higher.

There was a TV show called **House, MD,** a medical drama that originally ran on FOX for eight seasons, from 2004, to 2012. I loved that show. House was fond of saying, *"everybody lies."* According to House, it's a basic truth of the human condition. The only variable is about what. That's why I'm suspect of all the pharmaceutical advertising and research, no matter what their source: Medical Journals, Universities, CNN, print ads, or the FDA. Most ads spend more time recanting, detracting, or disclosing their fine print and serious side effects.

Let me ask you. How do you feel about yourself at this very moment? Are you comfortable in your own body, or do you skirt friends, family, and acquaintances like a herpes lone wolf or leper? Unlike an off-ramp beggar, do you still have hope? Are you constantly on a *"Lysine"* retreat, but trapped in an *"Arginine"* M&M, peanut butter Reese's recurring nightmare? Remember, the number or severity of herpes outbreaks does not determine your self-worth. Life does not make mistakes. It's only our Ego that points its *"iatrogenic"* accusing finger at us.

Be still and know. We are an incredible creation of the Divine Universe. Not an iPhone, texting, twittering, neurotic, obsessive, stressed, itchy doppelganger. Women and men, young and old, who've been branded with the Scarlett "H" have a tremendous amount of pressure put on them by society when it comes to their HSV disease. It's understandable. How many selfies have you seen of a bald, pink, crusted, oozing penis, or a painful, bleeding, itchy vagina, taken on a *"night out with friends?"* The classic *Hangover* line: "What happens in Vegas. Stays in Vegas. Except, of course, for herpes."

If we feel the media's portrayal is true, it's time to update our mindset so their lack of common sense doesn't bother us. If it's not true, step-on-up and out of the *"poor me"* mind-shaft and into greener pastures. But please, get over it. Enjoy life, no matter what. Transform the way you feel about being a victim of the sexual predator and build meaningful relationships, despite herpes' ubiquitous presence.

A. Bullets vs. Band-Aids

According to a recent article in *The New York Times,* growing distrust in the medical profession poses a threat to public health and safety. In 1966, more than 73% percent of Americans had great confidence in our medical professionals. More recently only **34%** percent do. https://bit.ly/3GO6DAO

1946: the federal government spent less than one-cent ($0.01) on Health Care for every one-dollar ($1) on defense.

1965: the year Medicare and Medicaid were enacted; it had risen to only three-and-half (3.5) cents on the dollar. And despite the large increases in military spending under the Reagan administration, that ratio stayed constant in the 1980s.

2023: http://bit.ly/2DM2kaQ the U.S. Government was projected to *spend $2.9 Trillion Dollars on Health and Welfare*, and only *1.1 Trillion on National Defense.* You don't have to be a genius to understand the difference between **one-penny ($0.01)** for healthcare, to almost three-dollars ($3) for every one-dollar ($1) spent on defense. We're talking exploitation, not inflation. And with so much distrust, why are we still *"asking our doctor?"*

The powers to be will do whatever it takes to keep us doing or going *"their"* way. It's up to us to keep the course or try a different direction. It's obvious to everyone that our healthcare system is not working. The question is, *"Why?"*

B. God Heals, Drugs Mask & Parade

There's never a suitable time to have an outbreak. But the first herpes eruption is often the worst. We're confused and fearful when we come across our first blisters. Then we see our doctor, do bloodwork, take Acyclovir, get better, and life goes on. But for some, that stops working. When the *"process stops working;"* when Acyclovir, Valtrex, and Famvir only make us feel worse; when we complain to our doctor that we're still getting outbreaks; when she suggests that maybe an antidepressant will help, because there's not much else she can do. Hinting we should just learn to live with, or *"get over"* it. It's time for the Hermes Protocol.

Reasons for recurrent genital eruptions:
1. Lifestyle choices,
2. Burnout (stress),
3. Magic bullet treatments,
4. Emotional conflict,
5. Genetics,
6. Environmental triggers,
7. Wrong doctors,
8. Wrong treatments,
9. Financial obstacles to treatments,
10. Father time and wearing out, and a
11. Compromised Immune System.

Western medicine is bipolar. We have the best technology anywhere. If you're involved in an accident, the ER (Emergency Department) will save your life, if possible. On the other hand, when treating chronic degenerative diseases or viral infections, it's a complete failure. The answer to this dilemma, by traditional medical standards, is for doctors to prescribe more medications to mask an ever-increasing list of symptoms. But healing occurs when we remove, not add, more toxin. If there is a magic cure, it starts with your knife and fork, and continues with sleeping patterns. Changing certain lifestyle habits is critical to eliminate outbreaks. *"In this age of tweets, texts, abbreviated thinking, people expect a magic pill for every chronic illness, to go on pretending that all is well."* RH

It's understandable to *"ask your doctor"* and want to be cured by a magic pill. The other option is more complex and requires participation, change, and accountability. There's an old saying, *"You are what you eat. And if you are what you eat, are you fast, cheap, and easy?"* In retrospect, I ate too much *marzipan* (sugar), and had far too many *"Rum-and-Cokes."* An eternal blister waiting to break out of a compromised immune system.

There is no magic pill or surgery for ignoring our health for decades. Those with a Godly influence recognize that committing a sin requires penance. The word repent comes from the Greek word root *"to change."* Just as with spiritual repentance, if we constantly break out with herpes, we need physical and mental repentance. Genital Herpes doesn't care whether you're a black nurse, an angry white UPS driver, Donald, or Hillary, sick or healthy, rich or poor, fat or thin, vegetarian or meat eater, German or Chinese, vegetable or mineral, old or young, educated or illiterate, promiscuous or abstinent, or ?? Take a lesson from herpes. Open your gateway to self-examination, transformation, and education into **better health**.

PART THREE: HEALING THE BODY

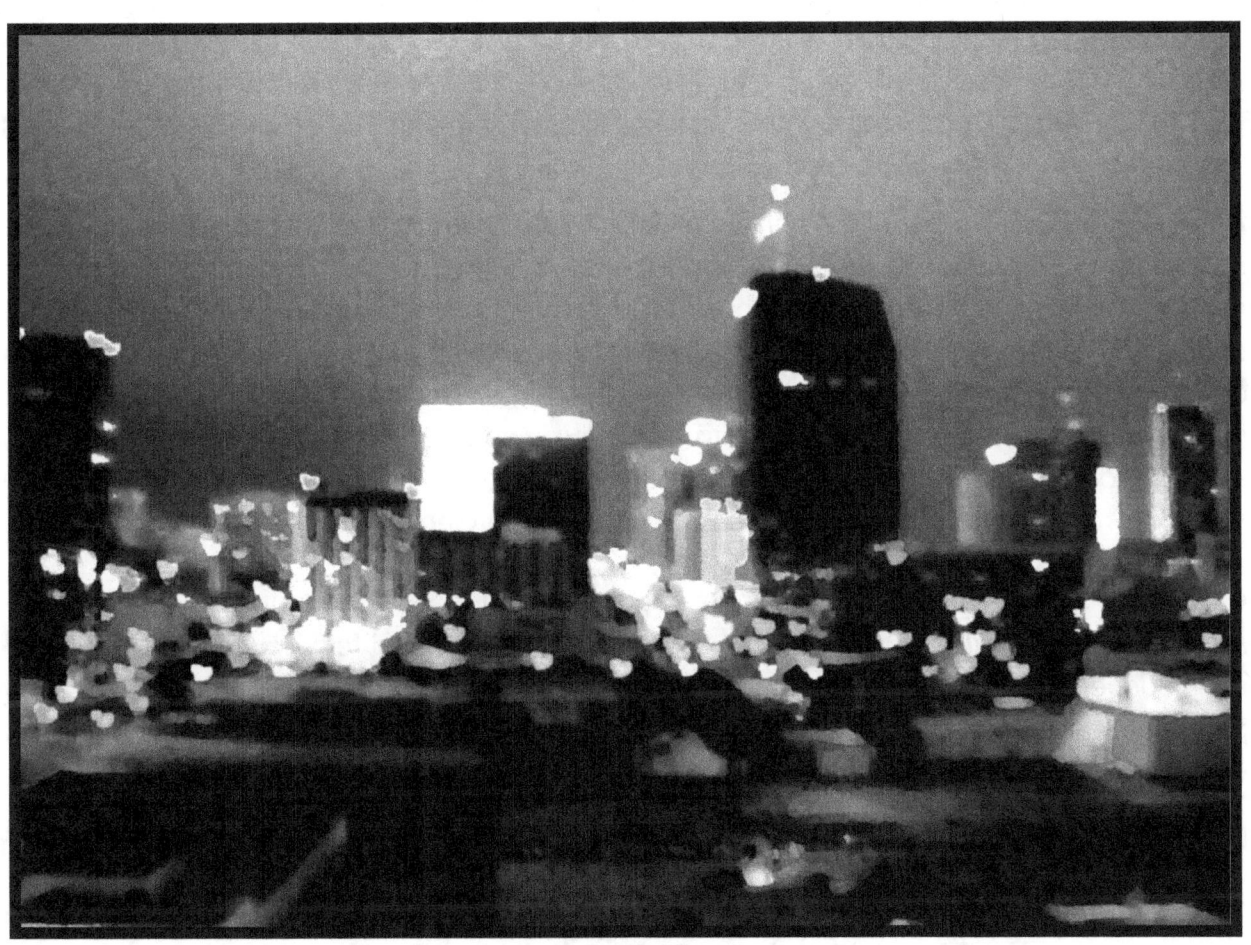

"City of Love"

Chapter 7: Pillars of Health

"You may choose to look the other way, but you can never say again that you did not know." - William Wilberforce

Miracle *"cures"* seldom resolve health issues but can injure savings accounts. Their focus is one-dimensional. As if there is only *"one"* aspect to health, the biological or physical component. Do they work? At times, but most often fall short. They can also complicate symptoms by incurring side effects that surface from the *"cure."* That was the author's experience with antiviral meds. As of April 2023, there was no herpes simplex virus (HSV) vaccine development news. The U.S. Food and Drug Administration (FDA) has not authorized any HSV vaccine.

As a reminder, *"You can't kill herpes inside the body by outside means, it can only be suppressed."* Even though there are *"promising strategies"* on the horizon, I'm not holding my breath. They've been hammering that nail for years. My heart wants to believe it. My mind says, *"shame on both of us."* Big Pharma has nothing to gain by galloping a vaccine or wonder drug through the stranglehold of clinical trials to *"heal"* herpes. It's not in their interest. Genital Herpes will continue to circle our wagon until we die. The only effective strategy to suppress herpes outbreaks (without toxic drugs) is to strengthen the immune system. That's the goal of the Hermes Protocol, to keep Genital Herpes dormant.

Not long ago: *"Where's my miracle?"* I began to wonder and thought, *"Maybe it's divine retribution for a reckless and confused life."* But, no matter how I felt, or what my *"negative"* mind suspected, the deeper Spiritual side never wavered. Difficulties are part of life. It's my job not to magnify or empower them. If they start to overwhelm me, I know what to do. You will, too, by the time you finish this book.

For many years I was focused and determined to find that magic *"silver-bullet."* Like a court order, directing Genital Herpes to cease and desist. Stop! No more out-breaks. But I never found an appellate court to rescind or reverse my herpes history. After decades in herpes purgatory, I'm outbreak free since 2017. Healing and remission occurred through the Hermes Protocol and four pillars of health. The goal is to stretch beyond the physical line of attack. To incorporate the mental, emotional, and spiritual realms that have a far greater influence on our physical health than we give them credit.

The Hermes Protocol: is designed to save time and frustration. When I refer to the *mind,* it includes the emotional, mental, and spiritual pillars of health, compared to the body's physical component. Even though the Hermes Protocol is 95% physical and only 5% invisible superglue, it's the glue that strengthens the immune system and our mind.

A. Four Pillars of Health

1. Physical
2. Emotional
3. Mental
4. Spiritual

The pillars of health are united in the Hermes Protocol through nutrition, diet, supplementation, lifestyle changes, mindfulness practices, detoxification, and alternative protocols. Given the right conditions, the body will maintain a state of dynamic equilibrium called *"good-health"* or *"well-being."* The remainder of this book will address the four pillars of health and how they balance the three adversaries to health.

Three Adversaries to Health

1. Deficiency
2. Toxicity
3. Uncontrolled mind

The Hermes Protocol: offers a variety of supplements and protocols to support the body's recovery from deficiency, toxicity, and an uncontrolled mind. Even though herpes outbreaks appear as a physical manifestation, they're intrinsically linked to all pillars. Yet we're lulled by America's medical profession into believing restoration of health is only a physical process, either through a pharmaceutical approach or surgery. But as a reminder, not one chronic disease has ever been healed using that method. As in zero. None. Granted, in an emergency situation we want immediate care to save our life, no matter what method. But not for chronic health conditions.

According to Wikipedia, http://bit.ly/2FofRI0 the U.S. in 2022 was ranked thirty-second (32) in men's mortality, with a life expectancy of seventy-seven (77) years, and women thirty-third (33), with a life expectancy of eighty-one-point-six (81.6) years. The irony, the United States spends exponentially more on health care than any other country in the world. Many, many times over. Also, of all the developed countries in the world, the U.S. has the highest *Infant Mortality Rate* http://bit.ly/2nhUStG.

August 19, 2017: a bit of disturbing news crossed the wires: *"First of Its Kind Survey Shows Vaccinated Children Get Sicker. The study concluded that vaccinated children were much more likely to be diagnosed with a chronic illness (including allergies and learning disabilities) compared to unvaccinated children. Vaccination increases have coincided with a rise in prevalence of dangerous chronic illness and NDDs."* http://bit.ly/2rKx0Uf

That should come as no surprise. Considering every disease in the U.S. has increased dramatically. For example, based on the current rate of autism, by 2025 *"Half the children born in the United States will be diagnosed with autism,"* according to Dr. Stephanie Seneff, a senior research scientist at the MIT Computer Science and Artificial Intelligence Laboratory. A study published in *JAMA* (2015), nearly 50% of adults living in the U.S. have diabetes or pre-diabetes.

The reason you bought this book is because of Genital Herpes. Health is important to you, as it is for most of us. Otherwise, why would we spend three times as much on sick care as any other developed country? And that doesn't include nutritional supplements. What do we get for that? Dismal and embarrassing results that keep getting worse. Whatever we've been doing is *"broken."* We need to change our approach. The Hermes Protocol can be such a change.

B. Three Undervalued Pillars

Beside the physical aspect of health, there are the Mental, Emotional, and Spiritual components. All intricately interrelated.

1. **Mental:** the ability to think through problems logically.
2. **Emotional:** the ability to feel what we and others are experiencing.
3. **Spiritual:** our soul, which is beyond thought and the mind.

When faced with not knowing the cause of a challenging and complicated illness like Genital Herpes, it's time to *"change"* our perception of the problem. Many find that difficult.

Sight is our most utilized sense of *"physical"* information. In terms of brain complexity, it's also the most developed. Visual-mental perceptions deeply influence memories. With our inherent negativity bias it's easy to gravitate toward anxiety when constantly focused on herpes outbreaks. To our astonishment, memory perceptions of what *"physically"* occurred in the past are often inaccurate. Especially in *"emotionally"* charged situations like herpes.

When we live by *"what-you-see-is-what-there-is,"* then physical reality is what you get. Life loses its charm and insightful emotional and spiritual component. It can still be valid and an *"efficient"* way to live, but Spirit is *"missing."* We all know the "by-the-numbers" type. They only follow the instructions mentality. There is a 'dead-zone' or detached feeling. As we all know from our dating experience, *"Looks can deceive: that's why perception and reality don't always match up."* Be mindful! The visual-physical-ego loves to trick not treat.

We are spiritual beings: with human, emotional, mental, and physical experiences. The mind is the repository of our beliefs, thoughts, emotions, and desires. The Spirit undergoes them. Spirituality is the basis of our existence. It manifests as thinking, sensations, emotions, and our physical bodies. That's why *"The doctor gets paid, while Spirit heals."*

All human beings have the same basic desire for happiness and to avoid pain. It's the ability to use our mind to fulfill those desires that's important. To be able to judge and learn from our mistakes. To consider the ramifications between the long and short-term consequences of our actions.

Happy and calm: physical discomforts such as pain and Genital Herpes can often be ignored. However, when we're angry or disturbed, even the best of circumstances, friends and family, money, or status, cannot make us happy. This suggests no matter how powerful our sensory or physical experiences appear to be, they cannot overwhelm the state of our mind. It's in the mental realm of happiness and pain that the application of the mind performs its most beneficial role.

The mind itself is neutral. It can be utilized in either in a destructive or constructive way. For example, much of our sufferings is the result of the mind's imagination to think into the future. It can create doubt, expectations, disappointments, and fear. That's why we emphasize the Psychology of Health to free ourselves from the chains and confines of mental outbreaks or breakdowns until we experience freedom.

"Use the best of both worlds, conventional and alternative medicine.
It's your greatest likelihood for a healthy outcome."
- Author Unknown

1. **Mental:** even though a healthy diet is vital, it's like sitting on a one-legged stool. It works for circus performers and acrobatic chefs. There is no magic or *"Hi-Ho Silver Bullet, herpes… away!"* Everybody's support system needs to harmonize to protect the body from infections. The body-mind connection is one more example of that. While the expression *"It's all in your head"* may refer to one's mental state, it doesn't diminish the physical symptoms that can arise from mental or emotional distress. People seem more willing to accept the mind/body connection to back pain than they are to herpes. That said, there is little dispute that stress is detrimental to both. To the surprise of doctors and patients, accumulating research suggests that most chronic back pain is NOT the result of illness or injury http://bit.ly/2Bygztz. Study after study indicates back pain is caused by our thoughts, feelings, and resulting behaviors. Recent studies demonstrated that treatment aimed at our beliefs and attitudes alleviated back pain. We've come to understand, we're not just what we eat, or what we do, but also what we think. To protect your body, protect your mind. And vice versa.

Not all the news about herpes infections and the mind is benign. *"Persistent herpes infections may be associated with cognitive impairments,"* reports *Psychological Medicine* http://bit.ly/2Gqd9wI. Researchers have found herpes virus infections cause cognitive impairment during and after acute encephalitis. Herpes Simplex Encephalitis (HSE) is a viral infection of the central nervous system. Fifty percent of its victims are over fifty (50) years old.

2013: a University of Michigan study, HSV-1 has been linked to mental impairment throughout life. *"This study is a first step in establishing an association between these viruses and cognition across a range of ages in the U.S. population."* http://bit.ly/2rHykqE

More than one third of the U.S. population tests positive for the herpes virus by early childhood, most individuals are not symptomatic, *"If HSV-1 begins to have impact on cognitive function early in life, HSV-1 infection in childhood may have important consequences for educational attainment and social mobility across the lifespan."* Something to think about. Since many assume they're fortunate to only have cold sores and not genital sores.

> *"I found that there is only one thing that heals every problem, and that is to know how to love yourself."* - Louise Hay

August 30, 2017: Louise Hay, *"an incredible, loving, generous, hilarious, peaceful, determined soul, passed away peacefully in her sleep. In coincidence, she passed away on the same night that Wayne Dyer did, two years ago."* The irony yesterday was "National Grief Awareness" day, so I'm going to do some Tapping on loss and grief with a Nick Ortner video in remembrance of Louise Hay. And my personal on-going emotional skirmishes with loss, due to my divorce. *"Thank you, Louise."*

2. Emotional: the *Journal of Neuroanatomy*, http://bit.ly/2EhRupV microwave radiation from cell phones, Wi-Fi routers, and computers is associated with many neuropsychiatric disorders. *"Depression is anger turned inward, and a Limbic-cortical dysregulation, and monoamine imbalance."* In plain English. Please, be careful with your iPhone. Try not to hold it near your head. Anyone struggling with emotional issues related to anxiety or depression, limit your exposure to wireless technology. Turn Wi-Fi off at night and try not to carry your cellphone on your body. At home, keep portable home phones, cellphones, and other electric devices out of the bedroom, a long distance from your bed.

2017: suicide rates were at a thirty-year (30) high. Mental disorders are the second most common cause of disability. Prescription drug abuse and overdose deaths are a public health emergency. While opioid pain killers are among the most lethal, psychiatric drugs also take their toll. In 2013, anti-anxiety benzodiazepine drugs accounted for nearly one-third of prescription overdose deaths. Emotions can kill. Directly and indirectly.

If you suffer from frequent Genital Herpes outbreaks, your emotional response may include, *"depression, anguish, distress, anger, diminution of self-esteem and hostility toward the person that infected you."* Studies have suggested that emotional stress can lead to repeated Genital Herpes infection. These studies also found that stress and herpes outbreaks occurred simultaneously. Suggesting it was the outbreak that caused the stress, rather than stress causing outbreaks. http://bit.ly/2Fn6kuz

Stress and herpes seem to be joined at the hip. An important consideration when dealing with emotional side effects. According to WebMd.com, *"Managing stress in healthy ways may help reduce how often you have a Genital Herpes outbreak. Ongoing stress (lasting more than a week) seems to trigger outbreaks more than any other lifestyle factor."* http://wb.md/2EiGfgO

Tactics: to speed up the process adjusting to herpes outbreaks:

First, realize that it's normal to be emotionally stressed with herpes outbreaks. Give yourself time to adjust, and remember, it will get easier.

Second, Genital Herpes is like most infections can be managed.

Third, feeling emotionally isolated, find an internet support group. To start, call a close friend or the National CDC STI Hotline 1-800-232-4636 for COVID-19 or Genital Herpes and speak to a counselor. There are many online support groups which can help you cope https://www.supportgroups.com/herpes.

Also, do not assume anything. Herpes is often more mental than physical. It will not prevent anyone from being involved in a long-term relationship. There are millions of couples all over the world who deal with Genital Herpes every day, and they make it work. Remember, you're not alone.

Additional Steps: to managing your stress better.

Get sufficient sleep. The more rested, the better at handling stress. Most people need about eight hours of sleep every night to function normally.

Balance your diet. Eat plenty of veggies and limit sugary foods. Also cut back on caffeine and alcohol if overindulging.

Exercise in moderation is a great stress reliever.

Reach out. Being with people and having fun can help you to forget outbreaks for a while. It's not healthy to dwell on them every minute.

Relax be content. Yoga, EFT, and meditation can be soothing and healing.

Although persistent stress may lead to outbreaks, the little daily annoyances we face are not stressful enough to trigger herpes symptoms. However, there is one stress factor that can knock down the front door to your peace of mind. It can also be more hazardous to your health than herpes, smoking, or obesity. **It's called loneliness.** Often associated with Genital Herpes, loneliness should not be ignored for long. The Herpes Protocol addresses those feelings in detail later.

Here's what Dr. Mercola had to say about it. *"An estimated 42.6 million Americans over the age of forty-five suffer from chronic loneliness, and more than twenty-five percent (25%) of the U.S. population lives alone. Loneliness is associated with higher blood pressure and higher risk of heart disease, stroke, dementia, depression, and lower survival rates for breast cancer patients. It is more hazardous to your health than obesity, raising your risk of early death by as much as fifty percent (50%)."*

Take-home message: don't isolate because of Genital Herpes. It can be more damaging than the outbreaks themselves. According to the American Osteopathic Association, which commissioned the Harris Poll cited above, loneliness plays a role in many chronic health conditions. These include pain, drug or alcohol abuse, depression, increased risk for Alzheimer's disease, heart attacks, stroke, and lower survival rates for breast cancer patients. People who are lonely are also more likely to experience:

1. Higher levels of stress for more herpes outbreaks.
2. Poor sleep for more herpes outbreaks.
3. Increased inflammation for more herpes outbreaks; and
4. Reduced immune function, more herpes outbreaks.

Emotional-Physical Connection
It's truly overwhelming how our emotions can influence overall health and herpes outbreaks A powerful force that either bolsters or undermines the immune system and our well-being. Epigenetics believes environmental factors such as stress and diet directly influence our genetic expression. It is the expression of our genes, not the genes themselves that determines whether we develop certain diseases or age prematurely. Guess where the herpes virus hides out? Yes, in our genetic DNA. And if we are chronically lonely and in a state of persistent Genital Herpes outbreaks, our negative *"emotions"* will influence the expression of our genes and affect the risk of developing more diseases.

Don't isolate. With or without an active herpes outbreak. Here are some suggestions and strategies that can help overcome the struggles with loneliness and isolation:

1. **Join a club.** *Meetup.com* is an online source with a vast array of local clubs and get-togethers. http://bit.ly/2FrQvmp
2. **Learn a new skill.** Enroll in a class or take an educational course.

3. **Consider a digital cleanse.** If Social Media has overtaken your life, consider taking steps to meet *"real"* people in person. Research shows Facebook may be more harmful than helpful to emotional well-being.

4. **Use digital media.** Phone calls or text messages can be a lifeline. Examples of this include sending encouraging text messages to other people who are experiencing outbreaks and struggling with loneliness.

5. **Exercise with others.** Joining a fitness club can open opportunities to meet like-minded people while improving physical fitness.

6. **Do local coffee shops** to develop a sense of community.

7. **Volunteer** to increase social interactions.

8. **Adopt** a companion dog or cat who can provide unconditional love and comfort. Studies show owning a pet can help protect against loneliness, depression, and anxiety. https://www.petfinder.com is an excellent resource.

9. **As a last option,** move and/or change jobs. It's not the answer for everyone, but for some it may be worthwhile, if it brings you closer to longtime friends or family.

Then relax, take it easy, be content. One last thought and comment about the following platforms: *Facebook, YouTube, Twitter, Instagram, Snapchat, Reddit, Pinterest, and LinkedIn.* Take a break.

Like all addictions, momentary pleasures have a long-term dark side. Researchers found *"that people who used social media for more than 2 hours a day were twice as likely to feel socially isolated."* http://bit.ly/2GsMMX4 The body is also being poisoned by constant WIFI radiation, compromising the immune system, and intensifying herpes outbreaks. There are more solutions on how to overcome loneliness, finding peace, and enjoying happiness at the end of this book.

> *"Not everybody believes in a formal religion,*
> *but nearly all believe in forgiveness--*
> *even if only desiring it for themselves."* – RH

3. **Spiritual:** Dr. Wayne Dyer wrote a book, *"There's a Spiritual Solution to Every Problem"* http://amzn.to/2BBVJcJ is a book by Wayne Dyer that sums up what is often a neglected or forgotten pillar in Western Medicine, the spiritual aspect of health. When confronted with a physical problem like Genital Herpes, we often depend on our mind's intellect to solve our financial worries, divorce and/or relationship difficulties. In Wayne Dyer's book, he shows us that there is a more powerful spiritual force at our fingertips that contains the solution to most problems by learning how to *"...unplug from the material world and awaken to the divine within."*

Each chapter contains practical applications for applying spiritual teachings to everyday problems, including affirmations, writing exercises, and guided meditations. It's a book about self-awareness and *"Tapping"* into the *"healing energy"* within us. Wayne Dyer, *"The mind is the source of problems. Your heart holds the answers to solving them."*

The book begins with *"You have been looking the wrong way."* And as one reviewer put it, *"This encourages a change in thinking. To realize we are so much more than our bodies and minds. If you are ready for this book, it can change your life. I am very grateful to the author, Wayne Dyer, for his insights and knowledge. What a game changer for me."*

Physical quest for health and mission to *"kill"* Genital Herpes through traditional antiviral medications. And yes, it's effective, but its effect is like nuking Hiroshima. Sure, it's possible to try and annihilate the enemy. But it'll only go into hiding, and if we're not careful, we may also be *"shot-down."* Eventually, all wars end. After the peace, the enemy and **"herpes"** will still be there. Unless we killed everything. Including ourselves.

The irony about the *"Hiroshima"* method, most cancer patients don't die from their disease, but from the *"nuclear"* treatment that eradicates their immune system. The problem with this near-sighted vision, and draconian *"carpet-bombing-medication"* method? We end up having to rebuild an entire country, and/or our body from top-to-bottom, inside, and out. Like all wars, there are no winners. It's never been a smart way to live a healthy, spiritual, mindful, and peaceful life. Maybe there is another way.

Once we delve into each *"pillar"* and start exploring their strengths. We'll realize how important *"Spirit"* is in our quest to be herpes free. *"Spirituality"* encourages us to be tolerant and self-accepting of ourselves even in the face of herpes adversity. That alone can be enough to reduce stress levels to the point that outbreaks stop. As one reviewer of the *"Sacred Self"* put it, *"An excellent path to feeling like the person you are is all you'll ever need to be to make it all work."*

C. The Immune System

*"All the information in this book is for educational purposes only.
It is not intended to diagnose, treat, or cure any disease or health condition."*

German Freudian Department of Aggregation (GoFDA)

Six people infected with Genital Herpes can each respond in a unique way to the *"various"* components of the Hermes Protocol. As is true for most treatments, there's not *"one"* solution that fits all, whether the disease is general malaise or Genital Herpes. The Hermes Protocol is designed to account for those differences. There are various combinations and options to choose from that will start you on the road to recovery and put Genital Herpes back behind bars.

Most herpes sufferers have tried numerous so-called *"cures"* only to *"break-out"* in one disappointment and failure after another. The reason most miracle products seldom work or marginally at best, they address the body's dashboard *"herpes"* warning lights, which tells us there is a problem with the immune system. Taking the approach by fixing your warning lights, whether Genital Herpes or General Motors, is treating the symptom, not the cause. Filling a deflated tire with air that has a nail-hole won't get you far. Yes, we can suppress symptoms by turning off the dashboard warning lights. But it won't fix the flat. In fact, other more serious side effects may surface if we continue to drive with a flat, or worse, on the rims. Then we'd be forced to treat those symptoms. And on, and on, and on, ad-infinitum. Until you abandon the clunker on some desolate highway.

We need to look under the hood. Go deeper into the immune system, and the warning lights will go off by themselves. Regrettably, many people just want a pill or quick fix to treat their symptoms. I don't blame them. I was one myself. Being healthy in today's toxic environment is a conscious, and often difficult, decision. But it's a responsibility we accept to be **Herpes Free.**

Good Health is not a Birth Right, as any chronic sick person in pain will attest to. Health is our most-valuable asset, but we need to be held accountable. Learn to use simple preventative measures that are known to be good for us without deceiving ourselves or making addictive excuses. Generally, a blue or green light reflects a vehicle in good working order. But then there is that dreaded blinking red light. We've all seen it. It looks like a red herpes blister, which immediately conjures up thoughts of *"I hope I make it home?"* or *"I wonder how much that's going to cost?"* or *"Oh, no, not another water pump!"*

Yes, seeing red sacral bumps invariably gives us a shock. While dashboard warning lights are troubling, they are good reminders. Proper maintenance can prolong the life of a car or body. Taking care of our car or body starts by first understanding its warning lights and symbols. And, yes, we can always trade in our tired old car (like a worn-out relationship) for a new one if there are constant warning signs. But unlike a marriage or car, we can't trade ourselves in for a healthy new *"me"* just because herpes warning blisters are constantly flashing red.

The feeling of driving a brand-new F-150 is uplifting! Only green lights and symbols. Like having a youthful and healthy immune system that protects us from catching the flu from a lack of sleep when we've overindulged. Too bad our body is not equipped with a more obvious dashboard. It would signal us when we've compromised our health, or due for a diaper change. ***"STOP!"*** There is a flashing red light on your immune system's dashboard. Quick, look at the body's health manual. Oh, my gosh, it's saying, *"Danger, Phyllis Nonsweet, danger! If you eat all that sugar, you're going to alter the balance of your "gut-flora" and risk a systemic fungal infection."* If it were only that simple.

Five Immune Warning Signs:

1. Constantly Tired

Sometimes the car won't start in the morning. We need a push or jump start to get us going. This is a 21st Century epidemic. There are many potential causes for fatigue, some more harmless than others. But when we're constantly tired, it may be time to see Dr. Safe Wrench or Dr. Feelgood.

2. Frequent Infections

The car is running hot. The coolant light flickers on and off. You pull over and call Triple Health. Dr. Feelgood says it might be your hormones, and why you can't cool down after a treadmill walk. It could also be the reason for frequent herpes outbreaks, urinary tract and yeast infections, inflamed gums, persistent indigestion, and constipation. All potential warning signs of a compromised immune system.

3. Constantly Sick

Accidents happen. You hit a shopping cart in Costco's parking lot, or back into a pole at work. Everyone gets into accidents or gets sick occasionally. But if you're catching every cold or flu that says *"Hello,"* it may be a sign that your immune system is compromised. You may need a tune-up or lab work to make sure everything is okay.

4. Severe Allergies

As we age, our bodies, like automobiles, tend to rust. Particularly if we live in an area of high humidity and severe winters. Then breaking out in rust is not that unusual. Allergies can also be a normal response. The same watery eyes during pollen season is probably nothing to worry about. But new and severe allergies may be an early warning sign that the immune system is malfunctioning. http://bit.ly/2GrkEne

5. Too Long to Heal

Did you notice the newly repainted driver's side door is starting to rust again? Like the time you cut yourself and it turned into a *"Colloidal-Silver"* emergency. It took forever to scab and heal? A compromised immune system can lead to significant delays in the healing process even for minor injuries. http://bit.ly/2GsVaFN (Nights of Healing)

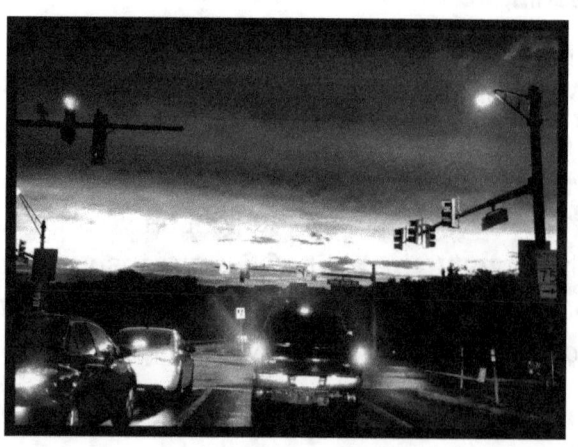

D. Sixteen Symptoms

WebMD.com: symptoms of potential immune problems: http://wb.md/2DM3I2y

1. Cold Hands,
2. Bathroom Problems,
3. Dry Eyes,
4. Fatigue,
5. Mild Fever,
6. Headaches,
7. Rashes (eczema, psoriasis, etc.),
8. Joints Ache,
9. Patchy Hair Loss,
10. Repeated Infections,
11. Sensitive to Sunlight,
12. Tingling or Numbness in Your Hands and Feet,
13. Trouble Swallowing,
14. Unexplained Weight Change,
15. White Patches, and
16. Yellowing of Your Skin or Eyes.

As good as our immune system can be, *it's not perfect.* If it kicks in too often, we can develop allergies, asthma, or eczema. If it turns on itself, instead of protecting us, we can develop autoimmune disorders like rheumatoid arthritis or diabetes. Keep in mind, these are only clues for immune complications. http://wb.md/2DX7SOK

The more informed we are as our own health advocates, the quicker we'll be able to figure out what's wrong. We used to think that the immune system kicks in only with an active outbreak. But new research suggests that it's in a constant struggle to contain the herpes virus. Apparently, herpes *"...produces copies of itself that leak into the skin every few days, not just every once-in-a-while."* In other words, our immune system is fighting Genital Herpes most of the time. Even without an active outbreak. https://tgam.ca/2nj3YGj

"Sometimes it loses the battle, but many times it's winning." I never considered or looked at it that way. It's certainly a more optimistic view than I had in the past. It's also why an infected person with a strong immune system, who is not symptomatic with an outbreak, can still infect their partner. Herpes viruses often leak through the skin in areas where they're not visible.

Current Herpes Antiviral Treatments: are limited and not always effective. Patients have choices, but antivirals must be taken on an ongoing basis to prevent outbreaks. If started after a lesion erupts, they shorten the infection duration, but not by much. The good news is that our immune system is constantly on guard, fighting to contain Genital Herpes. It's our job to find the right combination of protocols and tools to help it work even better; so, the virus remains fully contained.

E. Hormones and Herpes

Hormones affect every pillar of *"life,"* including the immune system and frequency of herpes outbreaks. Women can attest to that more so than men. Genital Herpes often coincides with their *"cycle."* Bloating, irritable mood, pelvic pain, or pressure are all common signs that a monthly period is coming soon. And for many women, this monthly guest often brings unwanted company, Genital Herpes.

Menses: to add offense to outbreaks, studies have confirmed that a women's menstrual period is one of the most common triggers for herpes outbreak. Stress is the most common. For some women, outbreaks start as a burning or tingling sensation. A numbness or pain in the genital area, vagina, vulva, or buttocks. Others experience swollen lymph nodes, fever, chills, and headaches. They may also feel pain or burning in one leg, the bottom of their foot.

Antivirals can almost always shorten an outbreak with early recognition and treatment. While menses can trigger herpes outbreaks, the opposite is not true. Menstrual periods do not change with herpes infections. Sometimes women have the misperception that their menstrual irregularities are related to Genital Herpes outbreaks. That is questionable. If you have an active outbreak and missed your period, or it's changed in some way, talk to your doctor. It's probably not related to herpes. Association is not always the cause.

For young women: a missed period can be normal, or it may be related to contraceptives. In some cases, it signals pregnancy. In the elderly, it can be part of perimenopause or menopause. Please contact your doctor to determine if you need to be evaluated. Herpes is often called a "silent" epidemic. The virus is easily transmitted from person to person with complete unawareness of its presence. Please, don't torture yourself trying to figure out who infected whom and when, or if your partner was unfaithful. Take a break. Herpes could have been dormant for months or even years. It's more constructive to work as a team to keep herpes at bay.

Financially strapped: go online. Many pharmaceutical companies, including GSK, the maker of Valtrex, have patient assistance programs for people who qualify. Also check out these websites:

1. **Medical Assistance Tool** https://medicineassistancetool.org/
2. **Pharmaceutical Patient Assistance Programs** www.rxassist.org
3. **Heart of the Pharmaceutical Industry** https://www.rxhope.com/ which keep lists of patient or drug assistance programs.

Shop around. Sometimes drug prices can vary by as much as sixty percent (60%). In general, chain pharmacies are more expensive than Walmart, Target, or warehouse clubs such as Costco. While they often require membership, in some states, membership isn't mandatory to use their pharmacy.

Your Thyroid: *"The Effects of Thyroid Hormone on HSV-1"* suggest that *"hormone imbalances may cause virus reactivation."* http://bit.ly/2DYSMZn

Do you want your health back? Are you ready to disable herpes infections? Regain lost energy and feel like a new self again? Then ask yourself, *"How important is my thyroid to my overall well-being and herpes outbreaks?"* In one word. Critical, indispensable, serious, key, vital, significant. Oops! I listed them *"one"* at-a-time. When the thyroid is not performing well, neither are you. It can create havoc in people's lives. Together with the adrenals, it's responsible for generating energy.

Your thyroid controls most every cell, tissue, and organ in the body. If it produces too much hormone, it's called hyperthyroidism. The body's systems speed up. To little thyroid, hypothyroidism, they slow down. Untreated thyroid disease leads to a myriad of conditions and diseases. Including heart disease, osteoporosis, infertility, and yes, "herpes reactivation." Research shows that there is also a strong genetic link between thyroid disease and autoimmune diseases, including diabetes, arthritis, and anemia.

Up to sixty percent of those with thyroid disease are unaware of their condition. Have your thyroid hormones checked by a health care specialist if you're cold when everyone else is warm. To find a good thyroid doctor, https://stopthethyroidmadness.com/ For an alternative medical doctor, try The American College for Advancement in Medicine. An association of integrative health practitioners. Go to www.acam.org, phone: 949-309-3520. Another option is The American Academy of Anti-Aging Medicine (A4M). They have doctors worldwide who are dedicated to preventive health.

The Adrenals: if the thyroid is the conductor for well-being, the adrenals are the orchestra. Both need to be reading from the same sheet music and playing in harmony. Otherwise, the composition, like the music of our health, will clatter, crunch, and tinkle. Overlooked causes of Adrenal Fatigue are chronic respiratory illnesses, and yes, herpes infections, predisposing people to chronic infections and respiratory problems.

Adrenal Fatigue, or Hypoadrenia symptoms include:

1. Autoimmune conditions,
2. Chronic fatigue (always feeling tired),
3. Brain fog,
4. Hormone imbalance,
5. Insulin resistance,
6. Lightheadedness,
7. Decreased sex drive/libido,
8. Moodiness and irritability,
9. Depression,
10. Muscle or bone loss,
11. Skin ailments,
12. Sleep disturbances,
13. Weight gain, and
14. Sweet and salty food cravings

"Adrenal Fatigue" was first coined in 1998 by Dr. James L. Wilson, a naturopath and chiropractor. His believed that chronic stress over time could affect the *"adrenals,"* thereby, producing inconsistent levels of cortisol in the blood stream. Sometimes too much, at other times not enough. You either feel *wired or tired*. Traditional medicine has no official diagnosis for Adrenal Fatigue. It considers a person to have either normal adrenal function or failure. In other words, black or white, nothing in between. *"Right."*

Adrenal Fatigue can occur after just one serious infection. Poorly performed dental procedures, such as a root canal, can also be a trigger. The more severe an infection, the more frequently it occurs. The longer it lasts, the more likely the adrenals are involved. It's not unusual for an infection to trigger an adrenal crisis. It can also take place over time.

Prolonged or recurrent herpes infections gradually weaken the adrenals and the body's immune system, making it even more difficult to fight off herpes infections. Other infectious agents, such as parasites and fungus are also common triggers. It's no surprise that Adrenal Fatigue and excessive tiredness are commonly associated with frequent herpes infections, including slower than normal healing times. Immune weakness from waning adrenals can set the stage for *fibromyalgia*, for even greater debilitation. If there is a longer than normal recovery period, decreased stamina, and unwarranted tiredness after an illness or infection, look to the adrenals.

Stress can trigger herpes outbreaks. Adequate adrenal support, a proper diet, healthy lifestyle, and effective stress management are key factors in minimizing stress-related herpes outbreaks. If we've been hypothyroid for several years, with or without being diagnosed, rest assured, the adrenals are working overtime just to keep us out of bed. They over-compensate with extra cortisol and adrenaline output. But in time, like any engine running at high RPMs, the engine conks out. It'll turn over but won't start. Not so different from our own health. Whether the stress is physical, mental, or emotional, they elicit a similar response from the adrenals. Our body's flight/fight stress response (high cortisol) is often depicted by *"Gronk"* the cave dweller deciding whether to run or fight the saber tooth tiger that's ready to make a burrito out of him.

Today the threat isn't *"real or in the flesh."* It's our iPhone *"imagery-addiction."* We're constantly running the one-hundred-yard dash (100-yard), from AM espressos to PM Wi-Fi tweets. To Bluetooth in-your-Face-book posts, to balancing an over-drawn checkbook. All the while *electro-magneting* ourselves with dangerous 5G and LTE radiation. Our thoughtless *"smart"* phone lifestyle is killing our pre-historic *"Gronk"* adrenals, who are trying their best to keep our engines running. The adrenals can only keep up with a high cortisol iPhone lifestyle for so long before they start to fail. Dysfunctional adrenals often manifest themselves in anxiety, light-headedness, shakiness, dizziness, racing heart, sudden weakness, nausea, or feeling hot.

Struggling adrenal symptoms are worth repeating:

1. Hard time falling asleep at night.
2. Waking up frequently during the night.
3. Slow to wake up in the morning, not feeling refreshed.
4. Bright lights irritate more than they should.
5. Sudden noises startle and disturb.
6. When standing from sitting, feeling lightheaded or dizzy.
7. Taking things too seriously and defensive.
8. Difficulty coping with certain people or events in life.

Self-test if you suspect Adrenal Fatigue:

TEST ONE: take and compare two blood pressure readings. One lying down and one standing. Rest five minutes lying down before taking your first reading. Stand up and immediately take another blood pressure reading. If the Blood Pressure (BP) is lower after standing, suspect reduced adrenal gland function. The degree to which the blood pressure drops when standing is often proportionate to the degree of dysfunction. Normal adrenal function elevates BP on standing to push blood to the brain. Test in the morning and evening since it's often normal one of the times.

TEST TWO: this is called the *"pupil test"* for levels of aldosterone, another adrenal hormone. A video http://bit.ly/2DY1Pts of how to test yourself.

TEST THREE: someone shine a bright light your way. If overly sensitive, uncomfortable with the bright light, it could be a sign of Adrenal Fatigue.

TEST FOUR: determine both thyroid and adrenal status with Daily Average Temperature readings. http://bit.ly/2rJHcfw

It's the 21st Century and we've misplaced our appreciation for simplicity. Many of us suffer from chronic Genital Herpes outbreaks because we're trying to create pleasure and comfort out of speed and urgency. We think in terms of efficiency rather than appreciation. Happiness and joy reduced, and satisfaction computerized. It's time to reconnect.

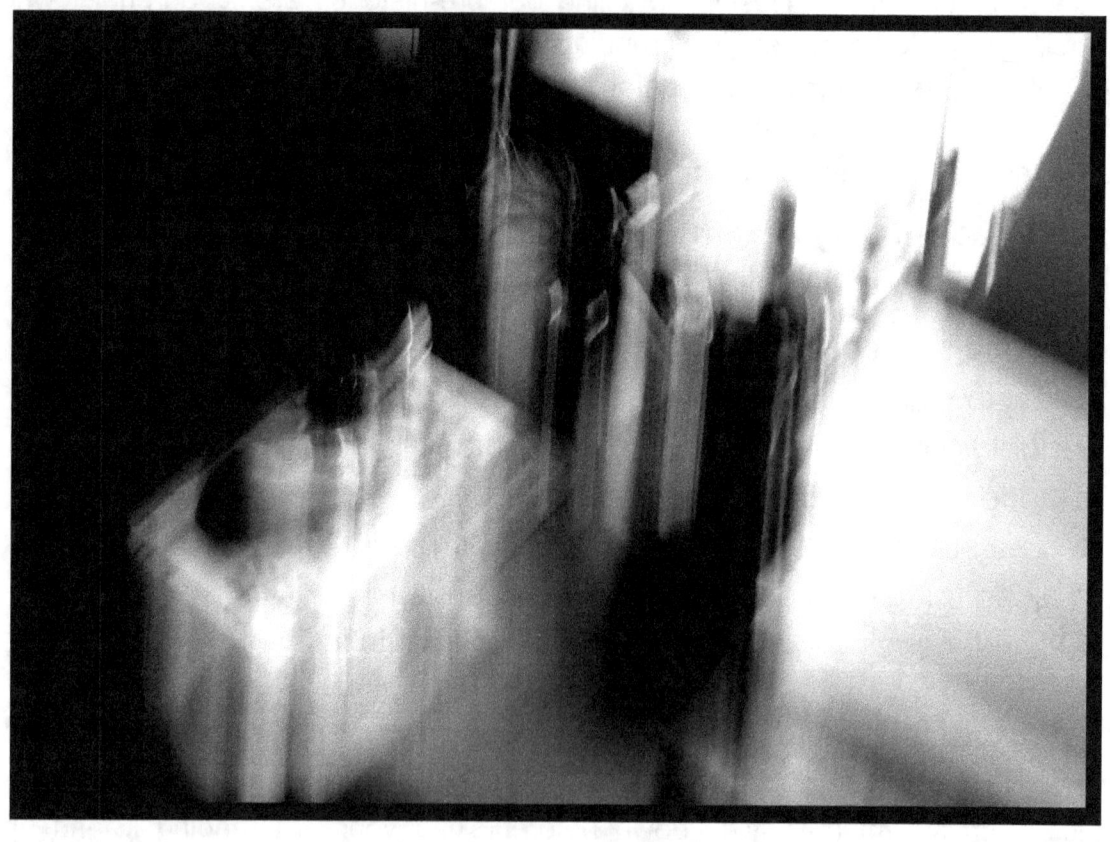

Chapter 8: Start Today

Start today to improve your health. Let go of anxiety and depression that binds us to sadness. The answers are simple, and they may surprise you. Three "physical" steps in the right direction:

1. **Eliminate** chlorinated faucet water and drink only natural, clean spring water.
2. **Add** minerals back into your diet, natural sea salt www.celticseasalt.com
3. **Purchase** ionic balanced trace minerals http://amzn.to/2FsPhau.

"The current IOM water recommendation for people ages 19 and older is drinking 3.7 liters (not quite a gallon) of pure, spring water for men and 2.7 liters (almost three quarts) for women. This is your overall fluid intake per day, including anything you eat or drink containing water such as fruits or vegetables. You may need to drink more if you live in a hot climate, exercise often, have a fever, or vomiting." http://bit.ly/2BBeEEG

Top priority: putting trace minerals back into our bodies. Our soil is so depleted that we receive a fraction of the nutritional value from just a few years ago. To know the body's existing vitamin and mineral levels, and for appropriate supplementation, do **a Hair Tissue Mineral Analysis (HTMA)**. When I got my results, I was shocked to learn how toxic and deficient my body was. HTMA tests can be done through Trace Elements, Inc., or Analytical Research Labs, Inc. Both reliable and accurate Labs.

1. HTMA kits can be ordered through Robert Thompson, M.D., 907-260-6914, who uses Trace Elements, Inc., or www.aurorahealthandnutrition.com.

2. Lawrence Wilson, M.D., who uses Analytical Research Labs, Inc. Dr. Wilson no longer consults personally but has a list of approved *"helpers"* to initiate his program. www.DrLWilson.com

On average, about 70% percent of our body weight is water. The remaining 30% to 40% percent are minerals. So, at 170 pounds, we carry 50 pounds of a life-giving soup of ionizing essential and trace minerals. From the more common calcium, magnesium, sodium, and potassium to the esoteric chromium, manganese, selenium, and copper. And the trace minerals, lithium, rubidium, cobalt, germanium, and molybdenum, just to name a few. Sea and rock salt contain minerals in the exact proportion that the body requires except for sodium. They are necessary for every single body function.

Dr. Charles Northern, a past leading scientist and researcher said, *"It's not commonly realized, however, that vitamins control the body's appropriation of minerals, and in the absence of minerals they have no function to perform. Lacking vitamins, the system can*

make some use of minerals, but lacking minerals, vitamins are useless." Decades later, Dr. Linus Pauling, winner of two Nobel prizes, said, *"You can trace every sickness, every disease and every ailment to a mineral deficiency."* Clearly their warnings have fallen on minerally depleted ears.

A. Forks and Knives

Now that you've started your engine, let's take a lap around the track. Then let's eat. Diet plays an important part in any therapy or protocol, including the Hermes Protocol. What's the old English proverb, *"Don't dig your grave with your own knife and fork."* But many of us do. *"I find that everyone is mineral-starved today, thanks to modern agricultural practices, stress and eating refined foods. Eating piles of cooked vegetables is the only way I know to obtain the nutrients everyone needs."* Dr. Lawrence Wilson

Let me forewarn. The *"Diet"* is restrictive, and not easy. Do your best. Remember the goal is to enhance the immune system to where it can keep herpes locked-up. Not only are most people mineral-starved, but their digestion is also weak. What we're not missing from our diets are chemicals. There are over three-thousand (3,000) chemicals permitted in food. Many damage or undermine our digestion and health. Organically grown food is best. Food from fast-food-restaurants is of inadequate quality and should be avoided.

DIET-IN-A-SHELL: Don't underestimate the power of nutrition and lifestyle to trump illness. If only we had more doctors who understood their importance and prescribed food choices instead of drugs. Diet is by and large "the" missing link in the health of our immune system and frequency of herpes outbreaks. Food over medicine and eating a plant-based diet is key in reclaiming good health. Plenty of "cooked" vegetables (not raw) with some animal protein each day.

Avoid all wheat, most fruits, and sugar. Keep meals simple. No more than two types of foods, and if you include dessert three types from proteins, carbs, and fats.

Today, processed foods are everywhere. Including your local gas station and pharmacy. Loaded with empty calories, they provide abundant, but insufficient nutritional rewards with no effort. So much so, that our brain declares, *"Don't stop eating!"* as biological hunger signals are overridden. In these days of twenty-four-seven 24/7 food availability, little exercise, and TV couch potato habits. *"Honey, can you get me some more Doritos?"* All it does is make us sick.

B. Healthy Food Choices

Focus on making healthy food and beverage choices to get the nutrients you need. Carbohydrates, protein, and fats are the three food groups that provide energy-producing nutrients. They can be broken down into: Grains, Vegetables, Fruits, Protein, Dairy, Oils, Solid Fats, and Added Sugars.

Recommendations to consider:
1. Eat plenty of cooked vegetables.
2. But not vegan or vegetarian.
3. Eat some animal protein daily.
4. For the first month avoid most fruit.
5. Instead, eat a few ounces of organic berries.
6. Keep meals down to two groups (Carbs, Protein, and/or Fat).
7. Portion size varies according to age, height, and lifestyle.
8. Eat slowly and chew food thoroughly.
9. Do not eat the same foods each day.
10. Try eating only natural, whole foods.
11. Starting do not eat powdered smoothies, or food bars.
12. Avoid drinking water with meals (some exceptions apply).
13. Organic food is best.
14. Avoid fast-food restaurants if possible; and
15. Shun all refined flour, junk food, and imitation or chemicalized food.

What's wrong with eating fruit?
1. Too high in sugar so it upsets the body's blood sugar.
2. Contains acids that can upset digestion.
3. Favors the growth of candida and other fungi.
4. Often sprayed with pesticides even when labeled organic.
5. Absorbs toxic potassium from N-P-K fertilizers.

Food Choices, Beverages, and Cooking Methods

Fruit: for the first month avoid all fruit except for a few olives, even though many are a reliable source of Lysine. This advice goes against many alternative nutritionists and doctors. From my own experience with Dr. Lawrence's eating plan? It works. Avoiding fruit can often reverse pre-type II diabetes and high blood sugar readings.

Simple Carbs: besides limiting fruit intake, AVOID all simple carbohydrates. This includes sugar, honey, maple syrup, agave syrup, fruit concentrate, dextrose, glucose, fructose, corn syrup, etc., etc., well, you get the Spartan and Teutonic message.

Protein: includes sardines, chicken, turkey, some lamb, or beef, but NO pork, ham, or bacon. Portion sizes for adults are four-to-five (4-5) ounces, no more than twice daily. Too much red meat, too much Arginine, spells *"outbreaks."*

Whole Grains: not recommended, but okay to have a small amount daily. Try organic blue corn tortilla chips, but try not to eat WHEAT, or products made with wheat.

Dairy: problematic for most people. They are either lactose intolerant or have a sensitivity to it. If we don't have the enzyme lactase, dairy doesn't get digested. This causes all sorts of unpleasantness, including explosive diarrhea and water retention. If dairy is OK for you, not a problem. Have up to six (6) ounces daily in the form of a quality *"organic"* yogurt or kefir. It's high in Lysine and helps keep herpes locked-up.

Vegetables: eat six-to-nine (6 to 9) cups of well-cooked vegetables each day. This is an important part of Hermes Protocol. Vegetables can include onions, shallots, leeks, garlic, carrots, radishes, Brussels sprouts, cauliflower, red cabbage, rutabaga, green beans, broccolini, and many, many more. Avoid nightshade vegetables (tomatoes, potatoes, eggplant, and all peppers). They are high in lectins, a substance produced in all plants as a natural pesticide. They are *"sticky"* molecules that tend to attach to the walls of our intestines, creating little gaps between the cells, which allows undigested food particles to escape into the blood stream, causing inflammation and a leaky gut.

Garlic: this powerful *"anti-candida-herpes"* food is like onions or shallots but in its own category. Sometimes before lunch, I'll do *"Garlic"* for prevention of Genital Herpes and candida. Suggested daily dose for prevention, one teaspoon of fresh minced *"raw"* garlic with *"raw"* honey, and two teaspoons at the first sign of a Genital Herpes outbreak or candida infection.

Cooking Methods: some prefer steamed vegetables, others a pressure-cooker, crock pot or stir frying. Avoid roasting or deep frying.

Beverages: drink water. Buying spring water in gallon jugs is fine. If you filter water, a carbon filter is adequate. Avoid reverse osmosis water. It lacks mineral content and is suspected of picking up plastic residue. Try not to count or substitute other beverages for your daily water intake. That doesn't mean you can't drink them; they just won't count. Enjoy a tasty cup of bone broth, an excellent source of protein. Fresh carrot or wheat grass juice are also excellent if not filled with preservatives.

Alcoholic Beverages: a glass of haughty wine for all the wannabes? It's one of the most contaminated alcoholic beverages, often polluted with arsenic even if labeled organic. Let me speak plainly, alcohol is bad for our health, even in moderation. http://cbsn.ws/2EnV1De

Until recently, science-backed wisdom said alcohol in moderation was good for our health. New scientific research says that there is no safe alcohol limit. It's linked to more than sixty different diseases, with one drink a day increasing the risk of breast cancer by four percent (4%). *"Responsible Drinking"* is a 21st-century mantra, but when it comes to cancer no amount of alcohol is safe.

Sugary Beverages: just say "NO" to all sugary drinks; sodas, diet sodas, Kool-Aid, Gatorade, Recharge, and most energy drinks.

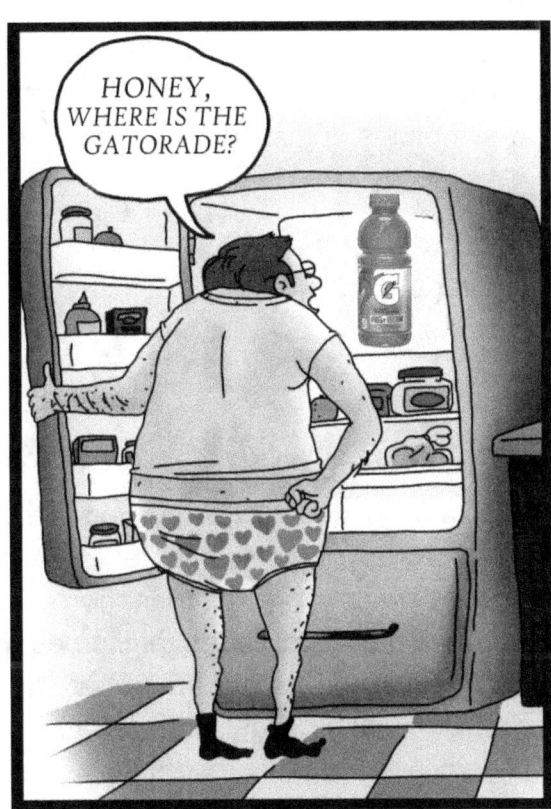

C. Nutrition for Herpes

The Do's: a diet high in Lysine helps control herpes outbreaks. Lysine is an amino acid that also strengthens the immune system to fight the virus.

Lysine-rich Foods:

1. **Fermented foods** like sauerkraut, miso, kefir, and organic yogurt.
2. **Add sea salt** to meals after cooking, a source of minerals.
3. **Broccoli,** Brussel sprouts and cauliflower, our *"best"* friends for herpes.

4. **Chicken, beef, lamb**, and sardines are rich in Lysine. (In moderation)

5. **Homemade yogurt** is rich in Lysine and probiotics. A daily serving of yogurt supports the herpes healing process; however, many *commercial* products contain gelatin or corn syrup that is high in Arginine, which can cause more outbreaks.

6. **Drinking water** improves the alkaline balance of the body. Avoid caffeinated drinks, as caffeine increases Arginine levels.

7. **Coconut oil** is an excellent source of medium chain triglycerides. Its lauric and caprylic acid also have antiviral effects.

Bon-Appetite: the frequency and symptoms of Genital Herpes can vary depending on the strength of a person's immune system. A nourishing diet strengthens immune function and why some people don't show symptoms of the virus.

Improve Immune Function:
1. Eat a *"healing-diet"* low in processed foods.
2. Avoid smoking or using drugs.
3. Exercise regularly, but moderately.
4. Manage stress.
5. Get seven to eight (7 to 8) hours of sleep a night.
6. Limit your exposure to toxic chemicals, like bromine and chlorine.

A comprehensive nutritional balancing program is a good start to keep Genital Herpes dormant. Meanwhile, *"bon-appetite,"* enjoy your steamed cauliflower and broccoli. If you don't cook much, try *Joyful Cooking*, by Joy Feldman, *"nutritional balancing"* cookbook recommended by Dr. Wilson. Since the topic is Genital Herpes, nutrition is not covered in detail, but don't neglect its importance and impact on herpes. If you snack, try not to. The exception is diabetes and/or unstable blood sugar. In that case, some food between meals may be important. Try not to gorge on too many carbs; instead, have some protein with a small amount of fat. For those who do not like to cook, or travel often, eating in restaurants can work if you avoid fast food chains. They use too many additives or chemicals in their *"smiley-meals."*

The Don'ts: Arginine promotes the growth and replication of herpes. Eating Arginine rich foods may be okay on the condition the Arginine-Lysine ratio is in favor of Lysine. However, to be on the safe side of outbreaks, limit the following high-Arginine foods:

1. Seeds and nuts
2. No Coconuts. The oil is fine since it has no amino acids.
3. Orange juice
4. Chocolate
5. Wheat products, Oat, and Lentils.

6. Protein supplements
7. Gelatin
8. Citrulline found in watermelons.

Avoid most acidic foods and drinks They weaken the immune system:

1. Alcohol, Caffeine, and junk food.
2. Eating too much red meat.
3. All processed/white flour products.
4. Food additives, and
5. Artificial sweeteners.
6. Birthday Celebrations are the Exception. Enjoy!

1984: Uncle Alfred, Aunt Krista
Celebrating Oma's '80th Birthday

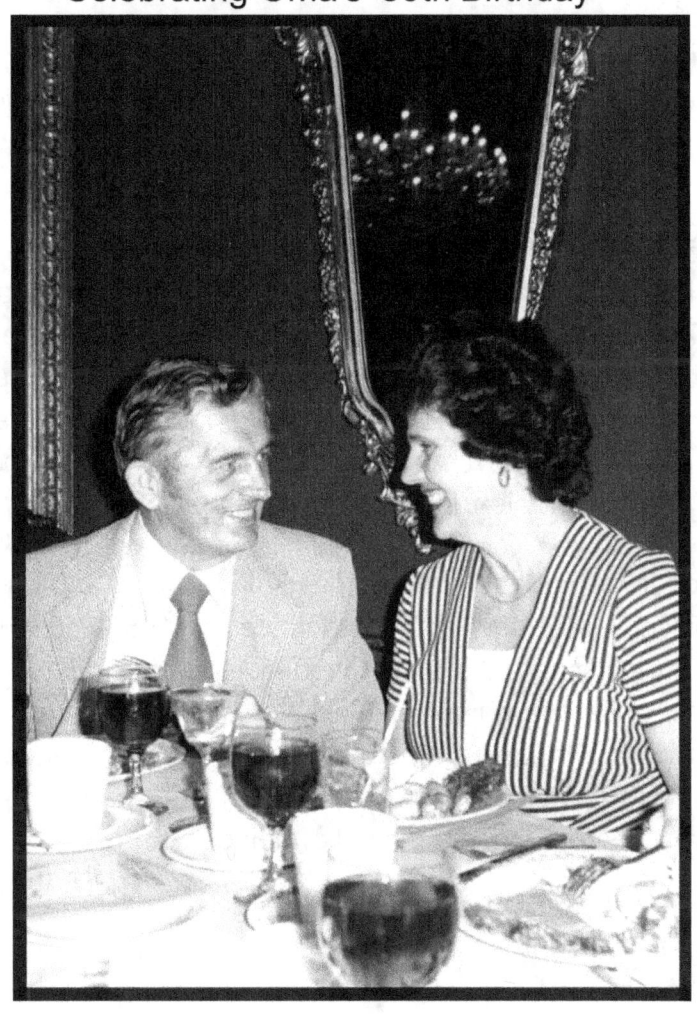

D. Chlorine-Fluoride-Bromine

Evil Threesomes: will undermine the immune system and can contribute to frequent Genital Herpes outbreaks.

1. Chlorine: adding chlorine to drinking water has saved millions of lives. It also comes at a great price. According to the U.S. Council of Environmental Quality, the cancer risk for people who drink chlorinated water is ninety-three percent (93%) higher than those who don't. It's also linked to heart attacks, reproductive problems, and damaged gut flora. When the gut flora is destroyed it disrupts digestion, causes bloating, and allows candida yeast to run rampant, further weakening the immune system,

Question: What's the difference between water chlorination and water fluoridation?

Chlorination is the process of adding chlorine (Cl2) to tap water. It kills certain bacteria and other microbes. It prevents the spread of waterborne diseases such as cholera, dysentery, typhoid etc.

Water fluoridation is the addition of fluoride to a public water supply for the *"mythical"* belief that it will reduce tooth decay. But scientists have known for years that it does nothing. In fact, it may do the opposite. According to a 2015 *Newsweek* article, *"There's hardly any evidence"* that the practice works. *"If anything, there may be some evidence the other way."* http://bit.ly/2DSBT2r

One thing we do know, both are cancer-agents and intentionally added to our nation's water supply with the full support of federal and state health agencies that are looking out for our health. The dangers posed by chlorine are even greater from bathing and showering. *"The amount of the carcinogenic compounds in chlorinated water absorbed by the skin is up to six-hundred percent (600%) higher than that absorbed from drinking chlorinated water."* Reduce the risk, install high-quality shower filter.

2. Fluoride: fluoride is a poison only surpassed in toxicity by arsenic. Yet it's routinely added to public drinking water and toothpaste since the 1950s. The EPA and other health agencies continue to insist that it's safe, despite mounting evidence of its health risks. **Fourteen countries** in Europe have outlawed the use of fluoride in drinking water. They regard it too toxic for public health. Yet the EPA and the American Dental Association (ADA) continue to claim fluoride is safe up to 4 ppm (four-parts-per-million), even though scientific studies prove its four times the level of being **unsafe.**

Protect your immune system:
1. Don't drink water straight out of the tap.
2. Invest in a shower filter.
3. Don't use toothpaste or other dental products that contain fluoride.

3. **Bromine:** is everywhere, and a significant issue in food and medicine. It has been implicated in thyroid disease, cancer, breast cysts, prostate inflammation, pancreatic dysfunction, ovarian hormonal dysfunction, and endometriosis. http://bit.ly/2nolOXK

What makes it dangerous? It competes for the same receptors used by iodine. To bromine, and the body cannot hold onto iodine, which affects every tissue in our body, but especially the thyroid. Bakers use bromated flour. It yields better dough and makes for a stronger, more elastic commercial product, at the expense of our wellbeing.

Bromine is found in:
1. Pesticides used on strawberries in California.
2. Plastics, like those found in computers.
3. Bakery goods.
4. Soft drinks; Mountain Dew, Gatorade, Squirt, Fresca, etc.
5. Brominated vegetable oils (BVOs).
6. Medications: Atrovent Inhaler, Atrovent Nasal Spray, Pro-Banthine (for ulcers).
7. Fire retardants used in fabrics, carpets, upholstery, and mattresses.

Our government is there to protect us. Wait a minute, is that true? In 1980 the U.S. Department of Agriculture (USDA) mandated the addition of bromine to flour, even though bromine causes apathy, decreased concentration, depression, headaches, irritability, delirium, schizophrenia, psychomotor retardation, and hallucinations. Oh, almost forgot, as well as endocrine disruption and cancers.

The antidote for bromine is increased iodine intake and sodium chloride (salt). The kidneys find it challenging to eliminate bromine when the body is deficient in salt. Bromine should be outlawed from all food, drinks, flour, jars, cans, bottles, and spas. Because of its toxicity in our food supply, consider supplementing with iodine. It may help to reduce the risk of at least five distinct types of cancer: breast, prostate, ovarian, thyroid, and pancreatic.

E. Hacking the Mind

"Processed food is addictive and promotes depression and early death," according to Dr. Robert Lustig and his book, *The Hacking of the American Mind: The Science Behind the Corporate Takeover of Our Bodies and Brains*. Dr. Mercola interviewed Dr. Lustig http://bit.ly/2DYimxy *about "how food companies and government policy deceived the American public and turned food into a weapon of self-destruction."* According to Dr. Lustig, *"Sugar, processed foods, and other addictive substances, as well as chronic use of social media, releases dopamine that fuels addiction and depletes serotonin, which fuels depression, and will prematurely kill you."*

But not before you have an endless string of herpes outbreaks and think about packing it in before you go on vacation. In his book Dr. Lustig talks about, *"if you want to be happy, raise your serotonin levels, not dopamine (pleasure). Four ways to increase serotonin, all are free."*

1. Making human connections.
2. Contributing to a larger cause.
3. Coping with stress (exercise and sleep).
4. Cooking real food.

"Eating real food that you prepare yourself is important." He emphasized the need for omega-3 fatty acids, especially DHA, a component of every cell in the body. More than 90% percent of the omega-3 fat in brain tissue is DHA. As it turns out, Facebook does not count as a 'human' connection. Social media generates dopamine, associated with pleasure. It drives addiction, not tryptophan and happiness. As dopamine goes up, serotonin and peace are flushed out. Online tweeting, texting, posting, surfing, and e-mailing are major sponsors for momentary pleasure but long-term misery.

What's the difference between pleasure and happiness?

Our grandparents had a much better understanding of happiness. To turn the trend of pleasure seeking, into happiness, understand their differences:

1. Pleasure is visceral; happiness is ethereal.
2. Pleasure is short-term; happiness long-term.
3. Pleasure is usually achieved alone, happiness in social settings.
4. Pleasure is taking; happiness giving.
5. Pleasure can be achieved with substances; happiness cannot.
6. Extreme pleasure often leads to addiction.
7. No such thing as being addicted to happiness.
8. Pleasure is dopamine; happiness serotonin.

The opioid crisis is looming wider and deeper across all demographics. Unless we understand the consequences of constantly seeking pleasure, as opposed to true happiness, many will be doomed to live in isolation, addiction, and constant discontent. Science doesn't get it. Businesses don't get it. The federal government is clueless. We, the people can get it, and then pray the *powers-to-be* will want to support us. I don't mean to sound pessimistic, but good luck to us all. **Dr. Lustig** said, *"There will be detractors who will say this is nonsense, but there are 600 references to demonstrate that this is not gobbledygook. The science actually predicted the phenomena that we see today and the society we've become."*

A simple food rule in deciding what to eat. *"If God didn't make it, don't eat it."* That includes any genetic tampering by Monsanto (now Bayer) or other industrial farming practices. Be careful here because the ego is smarter than our conscious mind. It tricks through perverted logic: *"God made the universe and all its atoms, so He made a SNICKERS bar?"*

Also, be suspect of *"packaged-foods,"* whether in a box, bottle, can, or wrapped in plastic. Avoid impulse snacks in the checkout line at your favorite grocery store or Starbucks. Most processed, packaged foods contain genetically modified ingredients, hydrogenated oils, and grains that provide little more than empty calories. Plus, you'll end up with more outbreaks, a bloated belly, and a starved immune system.

Diets Don't Work: cooking real foods does. A diet that promotes health and a strong immune system is high in beneficial fats (avocados), steamed veggies, moderate amount of high-quality protein, and low sugar consumption with a small amount of non-vegetable carbs (grains). We all know diets don't work. It's not news. The scenario goes like this. *"On average, in the first six months, people lose ten-to-fifteen (10-15) pounds, then their weight loss stalls for a bit, at which time they start gaining the weight back again."*

Foods That Don't Work

Unfermented soy: blocks the uptake of iodine to the thyroid, starving it of an essential nutrient. This means no tofu, soy milk, edamame, or soybean oil. Check labels. The oil is cheap and in limitless products.

Gluten: avoid it. It is mostly found in wheat, but also in other grains, including rye, barley, oats and spelt. Yes, oats, no matter what anyone says. Gluten is acidic, genetically modified, overproduced, full of empty calories. U.S. wheat contains three times the gluten than South American wheat. It can also cause immune antibody production in your thyroid.

Grains that contain gluten (*unfortunately some do, no matter what they say,*) have been linked to more than two-hundred (200) adverse health effects. In his book, *Grain Brain*, Dr. Perlmutter looked at gluten's neurological impact on the brain and autoimmune disease. He's certain that gluten sensitivity is involved in most chronic diseases, including deregulation of our immune system. According to Perlmutter, everyone is affected by gluten to some degree, even if we're not allergic.

Sugar: like its evil twin tobacco, tricked consumers into believing it isn't as bad as it is. Most people probably don't remember when *"the presidents and CEOs of the seven largest tobacco companies testified before Congress* http://bit.ly/2DZjQr6 *and said they did not believe nicotine was addictive."* To prove their point, in January 2014, Eric Lawson was the fifth **"Marlboro Man"** to ride the non-addictive tobacco train into an early grave. His death was linked to smoking. *Sugar,* the new *tobacco*.

2015: the award-winning documentary, *"Sugar-Coated,"* explores the dangers of sugar consumption and how it affects our health, the immune system and herpes outbreaks. The documentary makes a frightening comparison between people and ducks. It shows how sugar makes our livers fatty. Like a human *foie gras,* French for fatty liver. *Foie gras* is made from duck livers that have been fed copious amounts of sugar or carbs. Watch the Sugar-Coated trailer here: http://bit.ly/2BAWTFL

Dr. Mark Hyman, sugar http://bit.ly/2DW4MKV is eight times more addictive than cocaine. *One more time.* Sugar is eight times more addictive than cocaine. So, when my friends tell me they can't stop eating refined sugar, I understand why. But then try going to a 12th step meeting, like Overeaters Anonymous, but *stop*, or you may end up in a French restaurant as desert.

Dr. Hyman, *"The $1 trillion industrial food system is the biggest drug dealer around, responsible for contributing to tens of millions of deaths every year and siphoning trillions of dollars from our global economy through the loss of human and natural capital."* I've saved the last for worst. Up to forty (40) percent of U.S. healthcare expenditures are for diseases directly related to the overconsumption of sugar, mostly in the form of high fructose corn syrup (HFC). Some don't believe sugar is that bad. They think it just lacks micronutrients but otherwise harmless. Fifty years ago, Dr. Fredrick Stare, a prominent Harvard nutritionist, said the following (see seven comments below) about sugar and nutrition. His sugar-coated brain helped form government and public opinion for half a century: Life Extension, http://bit.ly/2EmBD9x

1. *Vitamin supplements are unnecessary for any normal, healthy person.*
2. *Sugar is an energy food. Put a teaspoon in your coffee.*
3. *Coca-Cola, a healthy between-meals snack.*
4. *Americans should drink a cup of corn oil a day.*
5. *We get as much food value from refined foods as natural foods.*
6. *Eat food additives. They're good for you.*
7. *White bread and brown bread are identical in food values.*

Annual Sugar Consumption, three-hundred (300) years:
1. **1700,** the average person consumed four (4) pounds of sugar per year.
2. **1800,** it had increased to eighteen (18) pounds of sugar per year.
3. **1900,** individual consumption rose to ninety (90) pounds of sugar per year.
4. **In 2009,** fifty (50%) percent of Americans consumed more than one-half (1/2) a pound of sugar **per day,** or one-hundred-eighty (180) pounds of sugar per year.

Afterthought: I eat little sugar. Maybe a few pounds a year. Somebody is eating more than three-hundred (300) pounds a year, or almost one pound of sugar a day. While grocery shopping the other day, I checked out what a pound of sugar looks and feels like. I got goosebumps. Either that, or my candida and the herpes clan anticipated a *Foie-Gras-Lovefest*. If you're eating a half a pound of sugar a day, like the average American, **please stop**. It may be all the immune system needs to be on the road to recovery and stop Genital Herpes outbreaks.

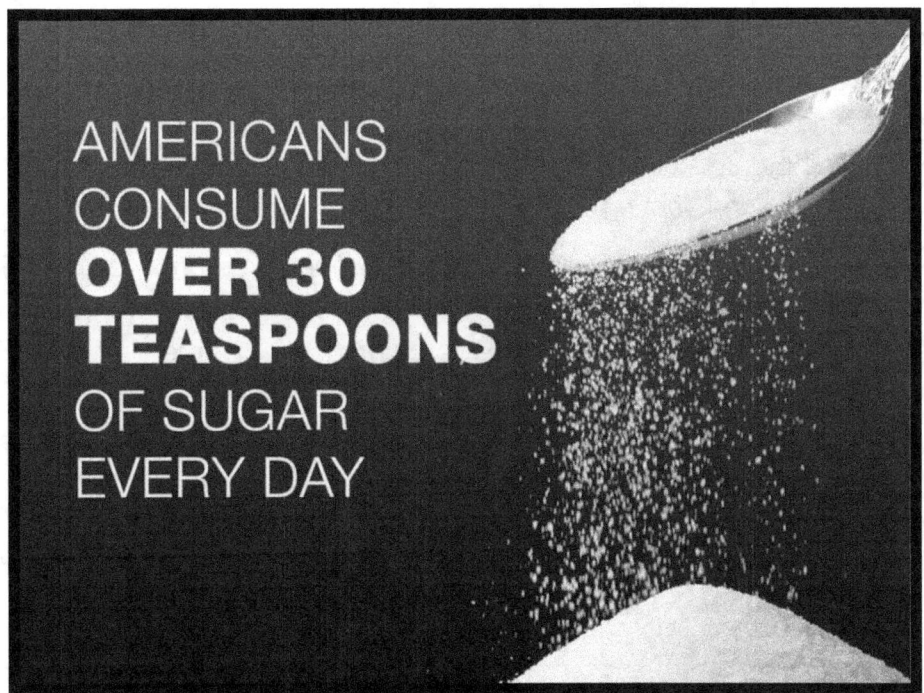

Chapter 9: Lifestyle Influences

Stress can become a way of life, but so can peace of mind, happiness, and living herpes free. However, reading about it will not make it so. It's a start, but the goal is to *"practice"* the Hermes Protocol.

Pain avoidance and pleasure seeking are common denominators for many Genital Herpes sufferers, while true happiness is elusive and rare. There always seems to be something or someone pushing our emotional *"red"* dashboard buttons, making us feel less than peaceful. According to Barbara Fredrickson, a psychologist and positive-emotions researcher, *"Most Americans have two positive experiences for every negative one."*

Barbara Fredrickson, *"To flourish emotionally, you need a three-to-one (3-to-1) ratio. Three positive emotions for every negative one. And only twenty (20%) percent of Americans fall into that category, which means eighty (80%) percent do not. Even worse, almost twenty-five (25%) percent of Americans experience no enjoyment at all!"* In our normal day-to-day life, we often allow ourselves to be dominated by negative emotions *(herpes)* and wishful-thinking *(herpes free)*. The Hermes Protocol reverses these patterns and prevents the influence of such thoughts and their emotions. In the process, we gain an emotional stability that eventually enters a peaceful state of mind and happiness.

A. Risk Factors

Supporting the immune system through a healthy diet, proper sleep, stress reduction, appropriate exercise, not smoking or drinking alcohol, can keep the *herpes predator* wishing and hoping that we relapse.

Herpes Risk Factors that can compromise the immune system:
1. Kissing someone with an active cold sore on the lips or eyes.
2. Engaging in any unprotected sex (oral, anal, vaginal, fingering, etc.).
3. Contact with viral secretions on other people's ulcers/sores.
4. Having illnesses that lower immune function, HIV/AIDS, or hepatitis.
5. Smoking.
6. Drinking too much alcohol.
7. Abusing prescription or non-prescription drugs.
8. Poor food choices (sugar) that exasperate herpes outbreaks.
9. Impaired Thymus Gland function.

Thymus: is the major gland of the immune system. Located below the thyroid and above the heart, its health determines the strength of our immune system. Chronic herpes infections are an indicator it may not be working properly. Correcting immune deficiencies (i.e., thyroid hormones) is essential, but may take time. Although lab tests are useful in verifying a compromised immune system, a history of repeated viral infections such as herpes, the flu or common cold is a good indicator. Repeated fungal infections in men and yeast infections in women can also hint at a compromised immune system and/or depressed thymus function.

Candida: is a fungal infection often found on the skin or mucous membranes (mouth). Under normal circumstances our immune system can defend against it; however, it's a formidable foe on steroids. If you have a history of sugar cravings and alcohol consumption they may be biologically influenced by candida, which is constantly on the alert for its next dose of carbohydrate, sugar, or high fructose corn syrup. It likes nothing better than a couple of shots of Jack, or a six-pack of Coors to proliferate and get pumped-up into a heavyweight nuisance. If you have a candida infection, your immune system is compromised.

2014 study at the University of Maryland measured the effects of drinking vodka on the immune system. *"Interestingly, the study showed that drinking alcohol caused an immediate rise in immune system activity. In fact, at the 5-hour stage, the levels of white blood cells were significantly lower, signaling a weaker immune system. Alcohol can have numerous negative effects on your body, reducing your body's capability to prevent Candida overgrowth."* https://bit.ly/3mb6ccN

If you are suffering from constant Genital Herpes outbreaks and Candida overgrowth, stay off the alcohol for now, and remember that it won't be forever. A 1995 study by Russian scientists showed http://bit.ly/2DJwGGE that Genital Herpes reduces immunity, and a 2008 Italian study showed that cold sores caused dysfunction of the immune response against candida. http://bit.ly/2DKl9ae So, who came first, **candida or herpes?** Either way, if the body is infected with herpes it has a reduced capacity to fight fungal infections, and herpes if afflicted with candida. Doug Kaufman, from *"Know the Cause"* https://knowthecause.com/ has an interesting perspective on *"Herpes."*

B. Sleep

Sleep deprivation mimics physical stress and suppresses immune function. So, after your third glass of wine *before* dinner, you decide to "bag" the chicken salad, and crunch-a-bunch of *'free & healthy'* peanuts, while polishing off the bottle of chardonnay. *Ouch!* You're asleep or passed out before your head hits the pillow. At 3:00 AM, like a bolt of lightning you wake up startled from a recurrent dream that you can't remember. What you do remember is the itch between your thighs before you went to bed.

Waking up early after a late night of drinking is common. It takes only a drink or two for alcohol to disrupt sleep patterns. Let's look at the difference between tipsy/drunk sleep and sober sleep, and why it's hard to sleep through a Vegas night out. As the alcohol wears off, the body enters REM sleep. Although the mind knows it needs more sleep, based on how it feels, the sympathetic nervous system (adrenals) is pushing us to wake us up to fix whatever is going on. Either that or to run like hell into a better state (fight or flight adrenals). Yes, the battle cry of the downtrodden and twelfth (12th) Step newcomers is: *"Life's unfair."* The solution for more shuteye after a night of drinking is to stop drinking.

Sleep Rejuvenates the immune system. While sleep requirements vary from person to person, most healthy adults need about seven-to-nine (7 to 9) hours of sleep a night to function at their best. Children and teens need more. Increasing sleep can result in decreased herpes outbreaks and/or often disappearing.

Ways to Improve the quality of your sleep:

1. Leave work at the office, the office at work.
2. After 8:00 PM turn cell phones OFF or airplane mode.
3. Avoid popping sleeping pills like Ambien, instead try melatonin.
4. Give the eyes and mind a chance to unwind.
5. "Wind down" an hour before going to bed/
6. Cut off electronic and media devices.
7. Sleep well.

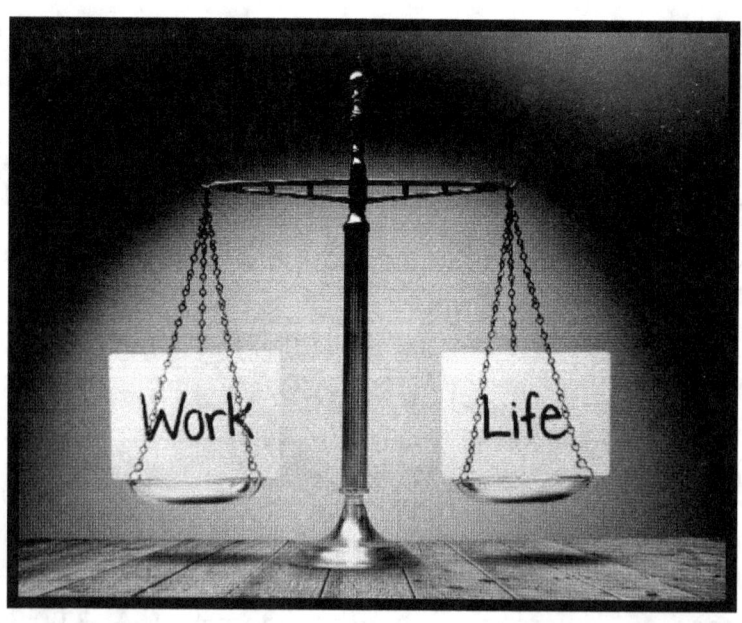

C. Stress

Orthodox medicine is still unclear why or how the herpes virus decides when to reactivate, but studies show that various forms of stress can be triggers. Minor stressful events and daily annoyances do not appear to be enough to trigger herpes symptoms; however, persistent stress leads to outbreaks. No matter what, managing stress can't hurt, but only help reduce Genital Herpes symptoms.

Stress Provoking Events:

1. **Common cold** can trigger oral herpes (HSV-1), no proof exists they trigger Genital Herpes (HSV-2).

2. **Hormonal changes** in women, like the menstrual cycle or pregnancy, can affect Genital Herpes outbreaks. Stress seems to be a contributing factor.

3. **Fatigue** is a form of physical stress, often caused by a lack of sleep.

4. **Immune suppression** caused by infections, steroid medications, or surgery.

5. **Overindulging** in alcohol, caffeine, and cigarettes.

6. **Vigorous sex** or friction to the skin during intercourse or masturbation.

7. **Excessive sweating** around the genital area from vigorous exercise.

8. **Exposure** to strong sunlight or ultraviolet light.

Stress Relieving Measures:

1. **Moderate** physical activity is a great stress reliever.

2. **Avoiding** emotional stress, such as depression or anxiety.

3. **Reaching out,** talking about your problems with those who care: a friend, family member, spouse, or therapist.

4. **Relax,** take it easy. Even a few minutes of downtime benefits. Relaxation techniques, such as yoga, biofeedback, meditation, and EFT (Emotional Freedom Technique) are beneficial.

5. **Quit** drinking and/or smoking. Tobacco and alcohol both increase blood pressure enough for herpes to maintain its potency.

D. Exercise

Exercise floods the body with feel-god endorphins that activate opiate receptors. They in turn reduce physical tension, alleviate stress, benefit depression, lighten anxiety, and facilitate sleep. **Yoga, Qigong,** and **Tai Chi** are uniquely effective at reducing stress because they combine exercise and meditation.

Regular exercise enhances the immune system, helping to prevent and fight herpes infections. It also supports heart disease, cancer, and osteoporosis. However, the intensity of exercise needs to be moderate to achieve this effect. Regular moderate exercise enhances, while strenuous, repetitive high-intensity exercise suppresses the immune system. To learn more how exercise effects immunity, http://bit.ly/2Fr2wsa.

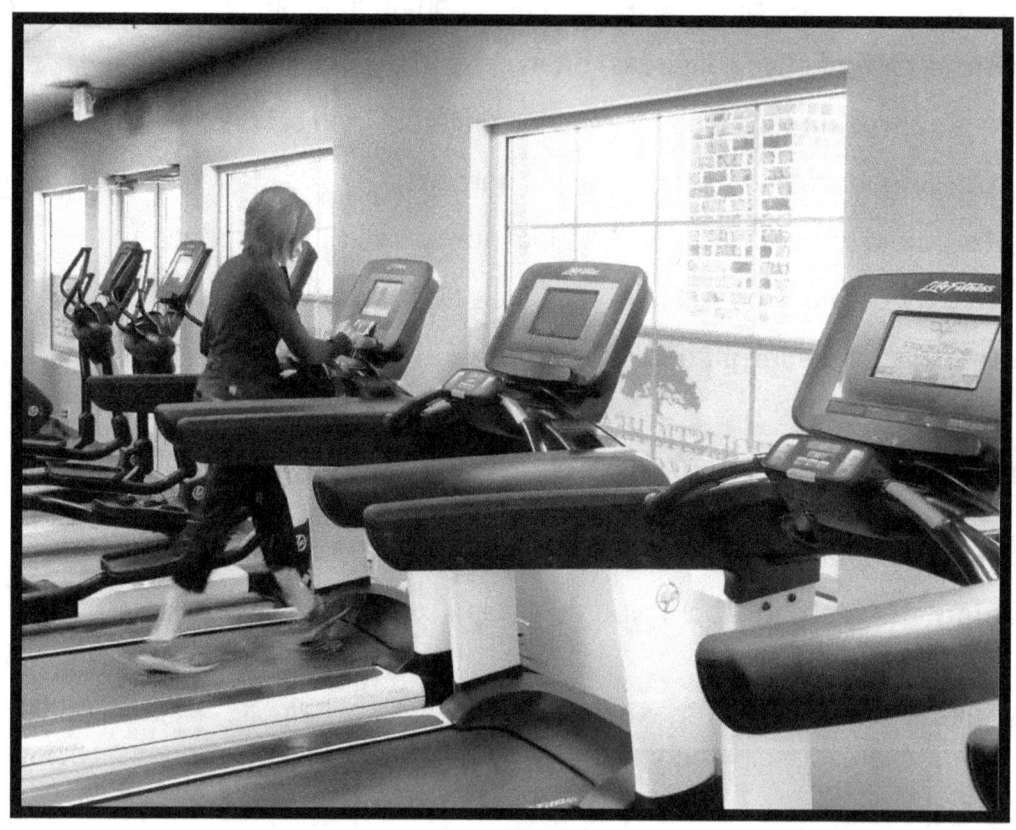

Exercise to Reduce Stress and Stay Healthy

E. Alcohol

The latest alcohol studies from the U.K. and Canada are sobering. A buzzkill, even for moderate drinkers. A glass of snooty wine a day was thought to keep the doctor away. Sorry, but even toasting to *"your health"* in moderation is an oxymoron.

The U.K.'s Department of Health now warns drinkers that consuming ANY amount of alcohol increases the risk to your health, including cancer and liver disease. I think I've drowned the alcohol subject into a blackout. I may have to attend a WOA meeting if I don't stop (Writers Overkill Anonymous).

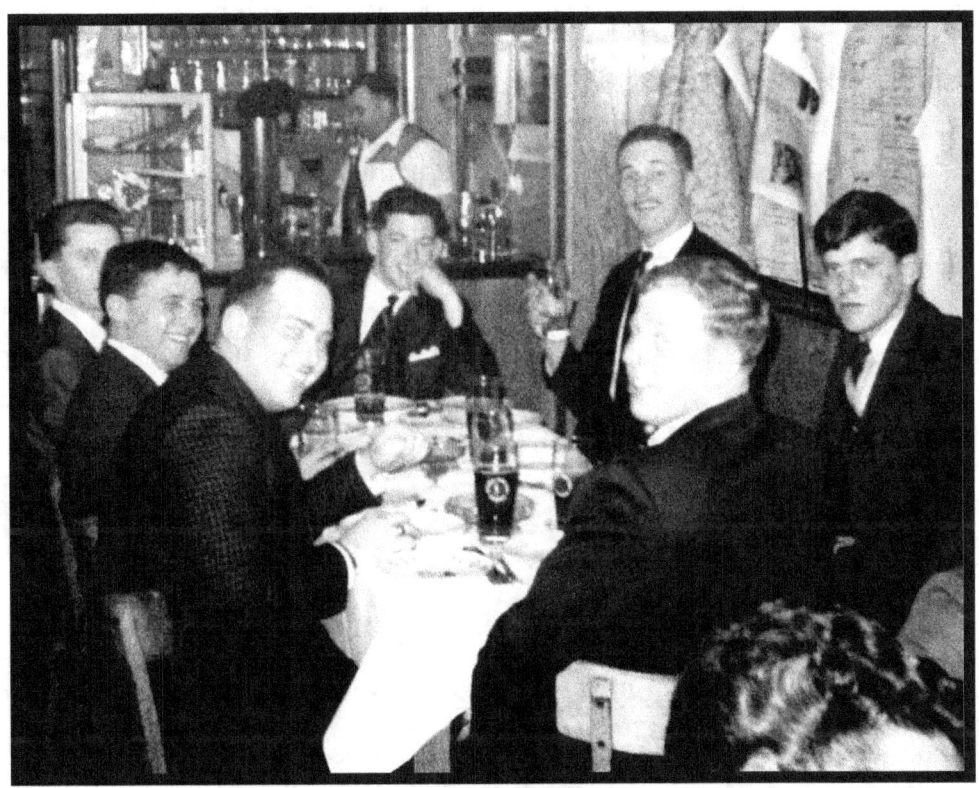

Rob's 1967 Wedding with U.S. Army Friends

Chapter 10: Protocols

Hermes Protocol for Genital Herpes is based on:

1. Clinical observations.
2. Diet and nutrition.
3. Psychological remedies.
4. Alternative protocols.
5. Immune support supplements.
6. Decreasing the body's toxicity load, and
7. Hair Tissue Mineral Analysis (HTMA). http://bit.ly/2GrdFdM

Physical Remedies support the immune system to suppress outbreaks, while **Psychological** remedies affect emotional and mental well-being. Combined, they are greater than the sum of their parts in gaining the upper hand against Genital Herpes. Never underestimate the power of the mind.

Familiarize yourself with each Physical and Psychological remedy to see which ones resonate with you. Be cautious before adding supplements without a Hair Tissue Mineral Analysis (HTMA). It may compromise an already imbalanced profile. Then consider your financial resources and determine what's affordable. HTMA results pinpoint obvious toxicity and deficiency issues. Follow recommendations based on your toxic load and nutritional-vitamin-mineral status.

HTMA Kits can be ordered through:

Robert Thompson, M.D., www.aurorahealthandnutrition.com, or

Lawrence Wilson, M.D. at www.DrLWilson.com, Analytical Research Labs, Inc.

Vitamin and mineral supplements are part of the Hermes Protocol. That and a proper diet are a good starting line. Not every protocol will work the same for everyone. Like fingerprints, we are unique in our constitution. Please review protocols and remedies in the next sections before making any decisions.

A. The Beck Protocol

Dr. Bob Beck developed the **Beck Protocol** from 1991 to 1997. It is an effective alternative course of action that supports the immune system and cleanses the body of infectious agents, including the herpes virus. **There are four steps** to the Beck Protocol:

1. The first step is Micro-Pulsing, or blood purification.
2. The second, Magnetic Pulsing.
3. The third is drinking colloidal silver; and
4. The fourth is drinking ozonated water.

The Beck Protocol reconciles a wide variety of health challenges. Watch Dr. Beck as he explains the *"Beck Protocol"* on YouTube. Enjoy this brilliant, compassionate genius who translated into plain words how electricity heals the body. http://bit.ly/2np6HOT Bob Beck at Granada Forum 1997

Because the herpes virus does not travel through the bloodstream, but along nerve fibers, it's difficult to treat. Any trauma to the nerves of the skin, such as a sunburn, a fever, or even the flu can trigger an outbreak. The Beck Protocol is recommended as a stand-alone protocol for Genital Herpes. If outbreaks continue after several weeks of treatment, there may be other factors compromising the immune system: lifestyle choices, systemic candida infection, or hormonal issues.

Step 1: Micro-Pulsing

Micro-Pulsing is zapping the blood with gentle electricity known as microcurrents. Bob Beck endorsed the Sota Silver Pulser as a **Micro-Pulser** for purifying the blood and making colloidal silver. Similar microcurrent devices, such as the TENS unit for pain relief or pacemakers for the heart, have been in use for decades. Microcurrents of electricity are considered safe.

Micro-Pulsing or Blood Purification mimics the body's own immune system. The University Hospital in Geneva discovered that white blood cells (leucocytes) kill pathogens by electrocuting them. They eject out an electronic flux focused on the bacterium via oxygen molecules: *"Zapp ZZssss"* and the bacterium dies. *Science & Vie Magazine*, Issue #972, September 1998. http://bit.ly/2FtMcqJ

Blood purification is safe and does not cause pain. Intensity levels can be adjusted, like a TENS unit, to an extremely comfortable *"pulsing"* tingle. If turned up too high, it may cause the muscles in the hand to twitch with each pulse. Simply lower the intensity.

Remarkable Discovery

In 1990, at the Albert Einstein College of Medicine, a small electrical current of fifty to one-hundred (50 to 100) MICRO amperes *"altered the outer protein layers of HIV virus in a petri dish so as to prevent its subsequent attachment to receptor sites."* (Science News, March 30, 1991, page 207.) Further research from Harvard and MIT showed that microcurrents eliminated viruses, parasites, fungi, bacteria, and pathogens in blood. http://bit.ly/2rNygGb

What's happened since 1990 with this ground-breaking invention? Not a thing. As in zero. The patent was sold, and nothing more came of it. I wonder if it has anything to do with being able to build your own microcurrent device for less than $100? Or buy it new from Sota Instruments for less than $300? https://bit.ly/3sZAVJS

Enter Bob Beck. Retired physicist and inventor, who researched electromedicine for most of his career. *"It occurred to me in a flash, why take the blood out of the body. Why not leave it in there where it belongs?"* Micro-Pulsing was born.

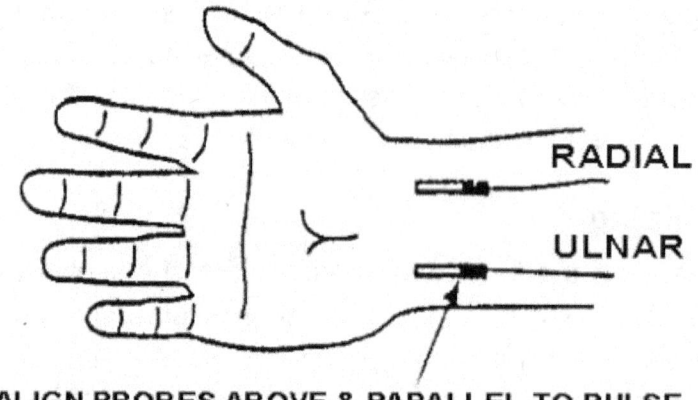

ALIGN PROBES ABOVE & PARALLEL TO PULSE

How to Micro-Pulse. Place two electrodes over the arteries on each side of the wrist. One over the radial artery on the thumb side, the other electrode over the ulnar artery, on the little finger side. Blood comes closer to the skin's surface at these pulse points. Start slowly. Build up from fifteen (15) minutes a day, to as long as two or three hours, depending on the severity of the infection. Micro-Pulsing accelerates the body's detoxification process. It's not unusual to experience flu-like detox symptoms. Back off if they are extreme.

Work your way up to a minimum of two hours a day, always backing off if detox symptoms become too severe. Bob Beck couldn't stress enough the importance of drinking plenty of fresh, clean water when Micro-Pulsing. It assists in eliminating toxins. Micro-Pulsing for Genital Herpes should be spread over a minimum of six weeks.

Occasionally, you still hear the myth and warnings about *electroporation*. Even Bob Beck warned about electroporation. But bloggers and apparently Bob Beck did not read the fine print of the research paper Bob often quoted.

The short answer *electroporation* does not apply to the Beck Protocol. It is a medical term used to increase the absorption of medications by also using electricity. Bob Beck assumed and warned that Micro-Pulsing would create electroporation. However, if you read the fine print it states that electroporation is based on an output *of two hundred volts per cm2*. The Bob Beck blood unit equates to only *about seven volts per cm2*. There's an enormous difference between two hundred volts per cm2, and seven volts per cm2. But that was Bob, he wanted to err on the side of caution.

Over the past twenty (20) years there have been no reports of any adverse effects attributed to electroporation, even from individuals who continued to use their medications while on the Beck Protocol. As a storyteller, Bob often talked about his garlic theory. As the years went by, he gradually embellished the effects of garlic from caution to demonizing, saying it was poison and that everyone should avoid it. The reality, most individuals have no problem eating garlic when using Beck technologies. Yes, some individuals are sensitive to garlic, but some are sensitive to strawberries. It doesn't make them poison. I love garlic. Maybe herpes is getting a taste of what it feels like being inside a crowded German bus with Garlic immigrants. Bob Beck endorsed the **Sota Silver Pulser** to also function as a Micro-Pulser for purifying the blood. For convenience, I use the Sota Silver Pulser for blood-purification and have a separate, stand-alone colloidal silver maker. There are several good units to choose from besides Sota. *The Micro-Particle Colloidal Silver Generator* from www.TheSilverEdge.com, or the **Silver Gen** colloidal generator from www.silvergen.com are both excellent units. If need more support, the advantage goes to the **Silver Edge.**

Step 2: Magnetic Pulsing

The SOTA Magnetic Pulser can be used anywhere on the body https://bit.ly/3Gx1USt. It immobilizes the herpes virus in the spine, root canals, the lymph system, the liver, and other organs. However, because the virus hides in nerve endings, blood purification alone will not deactivate them, but the Magnetic Pulser will. It's the second step of Bob Beck's Protocol. Once dislodged by the Magnetic Pulser they are a dead game. In case of an active outbreak, pulse the lesions for faster healing. The Magnetic Pulser offers the benefits of a pulsed magnetic field. It helps balance the body's natural electricity for improving immune function. While on the Bob Beck Protocol do not to use other alternative treatments for herpes.

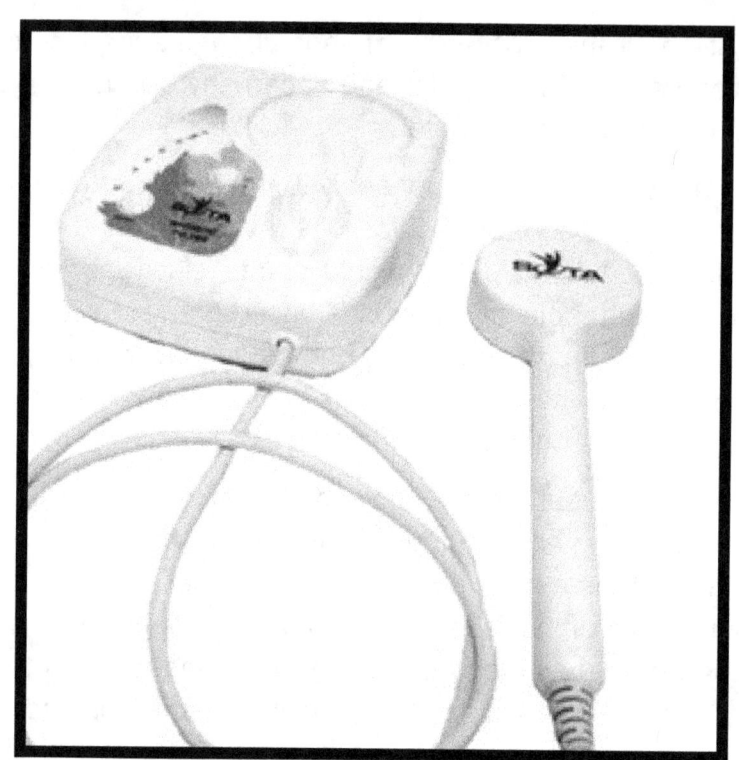

SOTA Magnetic Pulser

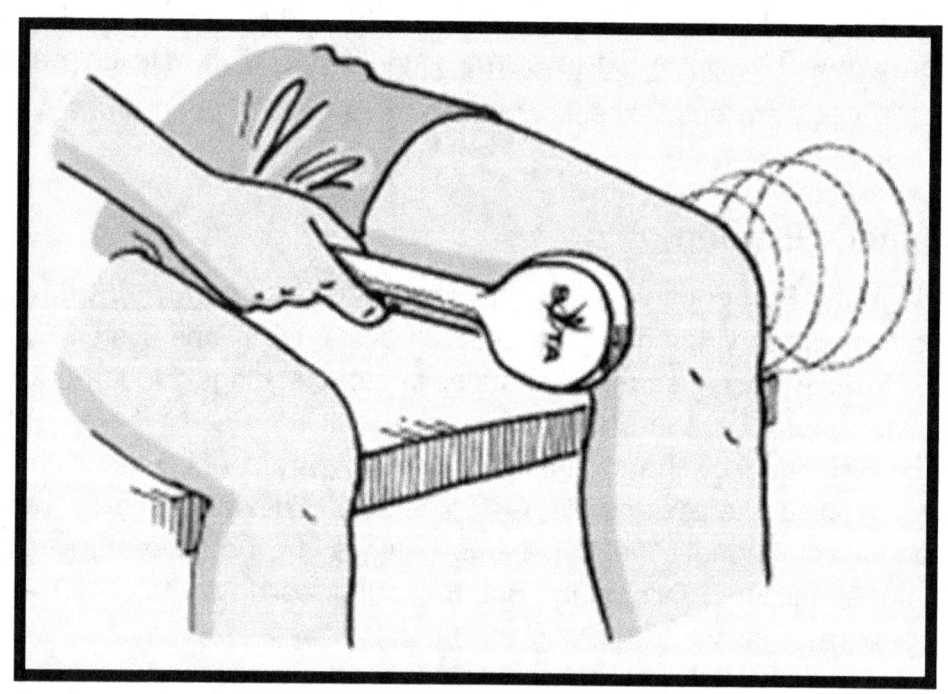

SOTA Magnetic Pulser

Step 3: Colloidal Silver

Bob Beck loved colloidal silver. He drank it like some people drink soda. With an active Genital Herpes outbreak, the author (Reinhard Hermes) consumed a half (1/2) ounce of 10 ppm home-made colloidal silver four-or-five (4 or 5) times a day for 14 days until the outbreak subsided. Hold the colloidal silver in your mouth, under the tongue, let it absorb sublingual, then swallow. Best on an empty stomach.

For Genital Herpes apply a 50/50 mixture of 99.99% *"liquid"* DMSO (Dimethyl Sulfoxide) and 25 ppm colloidal silver-gel to the blisters at the base of your spine and soles of the feet. The DMSO/silver solution is absorbed from the soles into the bloodstream. Start out with a lower DMSO concentration if there are any side effects. Test sensitivity by placing a few drops of 50% DMSO on your forearm.

Seventy percent (70%) DMSO gel is also available on Amazon to blend with either colloidal silver gel or liquid. Do the math yourself to get a 50% solution. For Genital Herpes at the base of the spine, apply the solution three times a day for 30 days, even if the infection has healed. Any area where DMSO is applied should be clean. DMSO has enhanced penetrating capabilities and can carry any contaminants into the surrounding tissue. Colloidal silver is an antimicrobial nutrient safe for humans, pets, and plants. Its target is to kill microbes, including any herpes virus circulating in the blood.

Question often asked: *"How much colloidal silver can I safely take each day?"* According to the Silver Safety Council (www.silversafety.org), the guidelines for safe consumption are as follows. The answer varies from person to person. Depending on body weight, overall health, and daily supplements. The Silver Safety Council's safe dosage levels are conservative and based on lifetime usage. Not in case of an infection. Remember, this is based on a *daily* colloidal silver safe dosage for the rest of your life, not randomly used to treat the flu or an infection.

First, multiply your body weight by twelve (12). Then divide that number by the ppm (parts per million) of the colloidal silver you're using. Twelve times your body weight, divided by the ppm of the colloidal silver = _____ the number of drops from an *eye dropper* you can ingest daily without harm.

1. **Weight**, 150 lbs., multiply 150 times 12, equals 1,800.
2. **Then divide** 1,800 by 10 ppm, or
3. **180 drops** of colloidal silver, or about a teaspoon a day.

If you watched any Bob Beck YouTube videos, it's obvious he consumed more than that for many years. He never incurred harm, only good health. If you're tall, weigh over two hundred pounds, the daily safe dosage will be two teaspoons (Silver Safety Council's conservative calculation).

Silver Safety Council's recommendations, I started with one teaspoon a day five ml (5 ml) of homemade ten ppm (10 ppm) colloidal silver. Then doubled the daily dose until I was consuming ten (10) teaspoons or 50 ml a day. It didn't stop the outbreaks but improved their severity and duration. Today, from a maintenance standpoint, I take two teaspoons (10 ml) a day, five days a week. Every couple of months I take a silver vacation and abstain for at least two months. Any amount above four teaspoons a day is regarded as therapeutic. To experiment with larger dosages, do so with caution.

Max Crarer, who wrote, **Everything You Need to Know About Colloidal Silver** http://amzn.to/2CpoiBBFJI5 said, *"I take over 150 mls, or ten tablespoons, a day and have experimented with that for a year with only beneficial effects, but what suits one may not help another."* Take "colloidal silver vacations" and abstain from using it at least for a month if there are no outbreaks. Do not try to push the body into any *"one"* supplement overuse. With one exception, lots of clean water. Regardless of the protocol, drink plenty of fresh water every day to flush out toxins, or any excess silver.

Jonathan Wright, MD: silver belongs to the family of metals that includes copper and gold, which also have health benefits when used properly. The primary concern in using these metals is that they'll accumulate in the body and lead to heavy metal toxicity. But if you have plenty of antioxidants in your diet, such as selenium, vitamin E, and amino acids like N-acetyl cysteine, you're most likely safe from any harmful effects. Germs, however, are not. **Dr. Wright** is not saying to take all the silver you want if you take plenty of antioxidants. What he means is that the body *requires* these antioxidants to eliminate silver from the body. Otherwise, there is a greater risk of silver accumulation, even at a normal daily dosage. Like most things in life, don't abuse colloidal silver.

Step 4: Ozonated Water

When Bob Beck started his protocol, there were only three parts. He added ozone after people complained of flu-like symptoms from die-off reactions of pathogens (herpes) killed during blood purification, the Pulser, and/or colloidal silver. It's called the **Herxheimer** effect. Sometimes the body is unable to expel toxins quickly enough, and that's why Bob stressed the importance of drinking plenty of clean water to support the body's detoxification channels, even before he added the ozone protocol.

After he discovered the book *Oxygen Therapies* by Ed McCabe, he added ozonated drinking water to the Beck Protocol. In a 1998 interview he explained why. *"Now we have a fourth approach... drinking ozonized water. Ozonated water helps reduce the toxins in the body. Ozone rapidly oxidizes and converts waste products long present in the body to water and carbon dioxide, which flush out easily and rapidly. Ozone is just like oxygen; it oxidizes waste products into water and carbon dioxide."*

Ozone is a great detoxifier, but back in the nineties ('90s) it was only available using expensive medical devices. So, what did Bob do? He built an inexpensive water-ozonator, so he could have a fresh glass of ozonated water at his convenience. And so, the fourth part of the Beck Protocol was born: drinking freshly ozonated water to help flush out toxins and oxygenate the blood. The other benefit? It kills pathogens, including the herpes virus.

Dr. Frank Shallenberger, MD, has authored a definitive book, *The Ozone Miracle,* accepted internationally as *"one of the world's most innovative and progressive medical professionals."* His website, www.theozonemiracle.com lists up-to-date ozone resources, free videos, and FAQs. Longevity Resources in Canada for reliable ozone generators. You can reach them at www.ozonegenerator.com or by calling toll free 1-877-543-3398 in the USA or Canada. For international callers 001-250-654-0092.

"But the only thing I ever hear about ozone… it's toxic and a pollutant, and there's a big hole in it over Antarctica." When combustion engines and factories release hydrocarbons into the atmosphere they interact with oxygen, nitrogen, and water vapor to yield SMOG! Negative health consequences of smog have to do with hydrocarbon, nitrate, peroxides, and Sulphur oxides, NOT ozone. Scientists just measure ozone to determine the level of the other pollutants.

What is the difference between medical ozone and that found in pollution? Medical grade is made from pure oxygen. Nothing else. Its therapy is one of the safest in the history of medicine. In the past thirty (30) years more than 2,500 papers on ozone's use have been published in peer reviewed scientific journals. Access many of these articles by going to the *American Academy of Ozone Therapy* at their web site www.aaot.us.

Best of all, ozone is toxic to all microbes, including bacteria, fungi, and viruses. Yes, even herpes. In today's age of super bugs and infections, ozone therapy can sometimes mean the difference between life and death. Ozone therapy is successful as a stand-alone remedy for chronic herpes infections. *"As with all viral infections, there is no cure in the sense that the virus is no longer present in the body. Therefore, I must emphasize that ozone therapy does not cure herpes infections in the sense that the virus is completely eradicated. However, it is excellent at inducing the cytokines that are very effective at decreasing viral replication."* Frank Shallenberger, MD, ***The Ozone Miracle***.

Ozonated drinking water is made by using a diffuser in distilled water and bubbling it for about 20 minutes. The ozone should be at 80-90 gamma. Once the water is ozonated it begins to lose ozone quickly. Drink it right away. If stored in a refrigerator it'll last 24 hours. If frozen, indefinitely.

Step 5: The Order of Things

Use the Magnetic Pulser before blood-purification. The Pulser dislodges pathogens like the herpes virus from lymph nodes, or any *"pulsed-gland,"* into the bloodstream. Blood purification then disables them. Remember, the Sota colloidal silver maker serves two functions: colloidal silver maker and Micro Pulser for blood purification.

Wait thirty minutes after using the Pulser before starting blood purification. They're NOT to be used at the same time. After finishing both electro-medicine procedures, wait another 15 to 30 minutes before taking colloidal silver. Electro-medicine *"opens"* the cells, then colloidal silver disables any unwanted microbe released into the bloodstream.

Common Side Effects

If there are a lot of toxins and pathogens in the body, the Beck Protocol will get their attention and they'll start looking for a more hospitable environment. To them you're now the HP Titanic, the Beck Protocol has given them an ultimatum: *"Jump ship or die."*

Since the skin is the body's largest elimination organ, rashes, pimples, and even boils with puss can develop. The locations vary, but the more distressing ones are on the face. This is not a bad sign; it just means that the Beck Protocol is working to kill herpes. If a person feels too sick, back off. Give the liver and kidneys a couple of days rest. Then start again with a smaller, slower, and longer build-up time. Don't overburden the liver and kidneys. Detoxification is not a 100-meter hurdle, but a marathon. There is conflicting information whether colloidal silver and ozonated water kill the *"good"* microbes in our intestinal tract. Error on the side of caution, add probiotics to nourish and replenish the *"friendly"* gut bacteria whenever using the Beck Protocol.

Daily Schedule after 5 PM

Weekends are more flexible. Remember, add a teaspoon of sea salt to any purified or spring water for the necessary electrolytes required by the Magnetic Pulser. Try to squeeze dinner in before drinking the allocated water, and/or before Blood Purification. Finish both electro-medicine treatments before taking supplements or colloidal silver.

- **5:00-PM -- Drink ozonated water,** with electrolytes.
- **5:30 PM – Drink more ozonated water,** with electrolytes.
- **6:00 PM – Start Magnetic Pulsing**
- **7:00 PM – Finish Magnetic Pulser**
- **7:00 PM – Start Blood Purification**
- **9:00 PM – Finish Blood Purifier**
- **9:30 PM – Drink Colloidal Silver** and take supplements.

B. Colloidal Silver

Colloidal silver is a favorite supplement for many, and I want to elaborate on its benefits, misperceptions, and as a stand-alone protocol. The internet *"gurus"* talk about how easy it is to make *"clean-and-pure"* colloidal silver. It's borrowed-big-box manufactured marketing hype. Making colloidal silver is not as easy as their *"plug-and-play"* propaganda want you to believe. It's not difficult, but it does take time and requires your attention. There are as many manufacturers as there are claims that theirs is the only *"pure"* and *"best"* colloidal silver on the market. More marketing duplicity.

"All products called ionic silver, colloidal silver, nano silver, hydrosol, or mild silver protein, are in fact just various forms of ionic silver. They all function by providing a delivery mechanism to release silver ions in the body. Otherwise, they would be useless." If you read or are told that one type of colloidal silver is better than the other, go to the Silver Safety Council's website to read their non-biased opinion. Also, when it comes to PPM or *'parts per million,'* there is no such thing as a *"safer"* level of PPM, just as there is no such thing as a more *"effective"* level of PPM. PPM is nothing more than a measure of how much water you're getting with silver. www.SilverSafety.org *Forbidden?* That's the error message from Google or Edge when I try to open the link. I wonder why?? Big Brother.

Particle size is not an indicator of safety or effectiveness. Keep colloidal silver away from sunlight and electrical and/or magnetic interference. TV's, microwaves, stoves, and fridges are bad companions for colloidal silver, as their magnetic fields cause silver particles to clump together.

There are thousands of personal internet testimonials of how colloidal silver improved every affliction known to man. But there are also well-known sites that warn consumers about silver's safety. Gee, I wonder what government body, or corporate behemoth, is behind that piece of propaganda? Here's a hint. In 1999 the FDA claimed that *"there is no scientific evidence to support the use of colloidal silver."* Conflicting information can be confusing. But when we look deeper into the naysayers *"scientific evidence,"* and their motivation, we find the same self-serving interests at work.

*"**Colloidal silver** is a completely natural, liquid mineral supplement found in almost every health food store in North America. It is much like mineral water, except that in this case, the only minerals in the water are tiny, sub-microscopic particles of pure silver. Pure silver, by itself, has been known for thousands of years to have powerful, broad-spectrum infection-fighting qualities. So, when the process for making colloidal silver was discovered in the late 1800s, shortly after Edison harnessed electricity, it immediately became a popular natural infection-fighting agent, used both topically on cuts, burns and infections, and internally as a remedy for a wide variety of infectious diseases."* **Life & Health Research Group, LLC.** http://bit.ly/2DOz7Ms

Benefits: Supported in the Medical Literature

Anti-Bacterial: colloidal silver's ability to control antibiotic-resistant superbugs is astonishing. UCLA Medical School documented over 650 different disease-causing pathogens that were destroyed in minutes when exposed to insignificant amounts of silver. Unlike antibiotics, it doesn't create resistance (to-date) in the *"bugs"* that it kills. That's a good thing, since we are at the end-stage of a serious antibiotic-resistant epidemic. In 2013 the (CDC) reported each year more than two-million people in the U.S. suffer because of antibiotic-resistant infections, and 23,000 of those die.

Antiviral: few will argue that colloidal silver is a powerful natural antibacterial and antifungal agent. But its ability to protect against viruses has not been embraced by the medical community until recently. June 2005: the journal, *Nanobiotechnology* published a 10-page study called *"Interaction of silver nanoparticles with HIV-1"* that demonstrated in test tubes that silver-nanoparticles inhibited the AIDS virus from binding to host cells. http://bit.ly/2noM1pb

When researchers placed the AIDS virus alongside human cells, silver particles stopped viral infection from taking place. In addition to HIV/AIDS, colloidal silver is an effective antiviral for pneumonia, herpes, shingles, warts, and against hepatitis C.

Even the Environmental Protection Agency (EPA) approved silver for certain antiviral purposes. According to the Silver Institute, **www.SilverInstitute.org**, the EPA approved Axen30 for use in day-care centers, schools, gymnasiums, and children's activity centers. Axen30 is a disinfectant formula consisting of 30-ppm silver. The EPA approved advertising claims to include:

1. **30-second kill time** on standard bacteria.
2. **2-minute kill time** on resistant bacteria MRSE and VRE.
3. **10-minute kill time** on fungi.
4. **30-second kill time** on HIV Type I.
5. **10-minute kill time** on other viruses.

Two respected researchers, Dr. Eric Gordon, MD and Dr. Kent Holtorf, MD, wrote in the *Townsend Letter for Doctors* that silver is most likely going to be *the* answer to any future global viral pandemic. *"A broad-spectrum antiviral agent that really works is needed to combat over 200 viruses that cause Upper Respiratory Tract Infections. Undoubtedly silver fits this bill."* All microbes, including viruses, need specific enzymes to help them live. Colloidal silver disables them, and therefore, Genital Herpes cannot survive. Colloidal silver is not a cure-all for herpes, but an effective treatment orally, topically, and as a rinse.

The Blues

Do you ever get the blues? Probably not like Paul Karason, or *"Papa Smurf,"* as he was affectionately called. Papa Smurf had a condition called *Argyria,* where a person's skin turns a greyish blue by over ingesting certain silver preparations. Colloidal silver did NOT cause this disorder, as many pharmaceutical Trojans, the media, or FDA watchdog proponents want you to believe. Infamously known as the *"blue-man,"* Paul Karason drank 700 ml, or almost three-fourths of a quart of silver a day before his skin turned blue. Yet it took fourteen (14) years. A rare individual among more than ten million users who've ever complained of a negative side effect. But it wasn't *colloidal* silver that turned him blue.

This is worth repeating: the *"blue-man"* effect was not caused by ingesting *colloidal* silver as is often misrepresented. Karason made his own silver mixture using **salts** to generate a **silver chloride solution** with large silver particles. This high-risk blend is far different from the colloidal silver solutions sold at stores or that you can make at home.

The *'Big-Bull-Shtick'* of Pig Farma. There has been a continuous, concentrated effort by drug companies to declare over-the-counter colloidal silver a *"threat to the environment."* They claim it has the potential to kill microorganisms that are *"ecologically important."* Well, at least they're concerned about killing microorganisms, although not humans, who *they* are killing. Let me translate *"ecologically,"* into *"economically"* important because it has the potential to kill their *"bottom-line,"* if people discover it could work for them at a fraction of the cost Big Pharma is charging.

In 2009 a coalition of environmentalists funded by major drug companies declared that nano-silver should be declared a *"pesticide."* It turned out *"not to be,"* but that doesn't mean it won't resurface. http://bit.ly/2nqtSr8 Fortunately, there is a way to make your own high-quality colloidal silver. Two good options are *The Micro Particle Colloidal Silver Generator* from www.TheSilverEdge.com or *The Silver Gen* colloidal generator from www.silvergen.com.

Wizard & Gwyneth: clinical studies on colloidal silver and its healing, infection-fighting benefits at http://bit.ly/2nqhVl9. TV's well-known Dr. Oz and Oscar-winning actor Gwyneth Paltrow have endorsed colloidal silver in this http://bit.ly/2rLG636 article. If you prefer videos, there are nearly twenty (20) brief instructional videos on making and using colloidal silver http://bit.ly/2rNEqpN.

CAUTION: individuals with kidney or liver disease may be at increased risk for developing silver toxicity. Drinking extra water helps eliminate silver and reduces its accumulation or risk of toxicity, which may also be increased if there is deficiency of selenium or vitamin E.

Homeopathy embraces a natural approach to the treatment of disease. Founded in Germany in the late 1700s, it's still practiced throughout Europe. Homeopathy literally means *"like-disease,"* and the prescribed medicine is *"like-the-disease"* expressed.

The homeopathic mantra, *"like cures like,"* compared to Western medicine's sacred repetition of *"drugs-radiation-and-surgery,"* or, to *"eliminate"* disease with a foreign or *"unrelated"* treatment. In homeopathy remedies are diluted and concentrated into mother tinctures of natural substances. Again-and-again the tincture or remedy is diluted, over-and-over again. With repeated dilution, the physical characteristics are diminished, but their energetic healing properties are actually increased. The higher the dilution, the more potent a remedy, and the greater its healing power. A contradiction to Western medicine's *"potency"* through strength philosophy.

The paradox of homeopathy is that the *"minimum-dose"* has the most medicinal effect and least amount of side effects. Homeopathy products are available in tablet, pellet, liquid, or oral spray forms.

Homeopathy also has a compelling safety history that includes children, pregnant and nursing women, and senior citizens. Side effects are rare but occur if too much of the correct remedy is used too frequently. Known as *"homeopathic aggravation,"* it's generally self-limiting, or can be relieved by drinking a strong cup of coffee. Which is something you don't want to do within a half-hour before or after taking a homeopathy remedy. It's also recommended that you do not eat or drink anything within that 30-minute window. A rule of thumb, the more acute and severe the symptoms, the more often the remedy is prescribed. In the initial stage, *"pellets"* are sometimes used every fifteen minutes, then tapered off as symptoms subside.

Homeopathic Remedy for Genital Herpes

Homeopathic remedies are tiny "pellets" of energy released when dissolved under the tongue. It's quite simple: pour the desired number of pellets into the cap and pop them under the tongue. Try not touch or handle the pellets directly. Some instructions recommend taking five to ten pellets, but often it's not necessary to take more than four or five. The number of pellets is not as important as the frequency of the dose. For example, with chronic Genital Herpes the length of treatment is more significant, whereas, in acute cases with severe symptoms the frequency is important.

Genital Herpes: I started with two homeopathic remedies and took two (2) pellets from each remedy twice a day. Another option is dissolving all eight (8) pellets the night before in a 12-ounce glass jar of *"clean"* water, then drinking the solution during the course of the next day on an empty stomach and/or at least thirty minutes prior or after eating. (*See Chapter 13, Section B*) At first, I was a bit confused trying to make sense of homeopathy's terminology. The internet is a haven for different and conflicting sources of information about dosage, forms, and potencies. After reading several books and researching www.joettecalabrese.com it became easier.

C. Cell Salts

Wilhelm H. Schuessler: another German doctor, in the late 1800s, discovered twelve (12) inorganic mineral salts after analyzing the *"ash-residue"* of human cells. He determined that numerous diseases are a deficiency or imbalance in these Cell-Salts, and with proper supplementation the body would heal itself.

Cell-Salts: are unique because they are absorbed by the mucous membranes (mouth) and not the body's digestive system. The irony is that many diseases have their origin in poor digestion. So, it doesn't matter whether you eat organic or GMO Happy Meals, or even supplement with the most natural, expensive vitamins. If your body can't digest or absorb their nutrients, it will continue to be in a state of deficiency and ill health.

Are you still hungry after eating a Big Whopper and fries? In a ground-breaking new study reported in the September 2017 issue of *Science Daily*, the brain can detect the nutrients (or lack of) in the food we eat. http://bit.ly/2nkDBA2 These are the same brain cells that control appetite. The University's School of Life Sciences *"discovered that brain cells called tanycytes, control energy levels and detect specific nutrients in the food we eat seconds after we eat them."*

Tanycytes respond to amino acids found in food, using the same tongue receptors that detect its flavor. When triggered, they send messages to the brain saying, *"I'm full. Thank you."* No wonder one super-sized bag of fries was never enough. My brain never got the message from my tanycytes. They never detected any real food.

That's not the case for *Cell-Salts, Tissue-Salts, Biochemic* cell salts, and Schuessler Salts. These are all different names for the same nourishing *'homeopathic'* preparations. Made from inorganic minerals, Cell-Salts can be taken without concern of toxicity, overdosing, or having an allergic reaction. In fact, Schuessler Salts are often used to treat allergies caused by mineral deficiencies or a defective metabolism. Cell Salts have a long history of safety and are known not to interfere with traditional medications. Remember, they're absorbed at the cell-level and not through digestion. They can also be added to a bottle of water bottle and sipped throughout the day. Best of all, they're child and *'Fido'* safe.

Cell-Salts are also less complicated than traditional homeopathy. There are only twelve basic salts, compared to several thousand homeopathic formulations. Since Dr. Schuessler's discovery, an additional fifteen salts have been verified; however, most treatments use the original twelve (12) salts. Schuessler salts are numbered from one to twelve, but American *'ego-nuity'* uses a different numbering system than the rest of the world. Not a big deal unless you're reading, learning, traveling, or ordering products from the rest of the world. Always double check *their names, **not their** numbers*.

If you have a physical issue, say muscle-cramps, simply google *"cell salts"* together with *"muscle-cramps."* It's easier than trying to memorize all their uses. There are also many reference books on Amazon.

For over 130 years, millions of people worldwide have used Cell-Salts. They have proved helpful in balancing many conditions, including Genital Herpes. Salts are an equilibrium remedy that balances the body's excess and/or deficiencies. They're often referred to as the *"vitamins & minerals"* of homeopathy. For supporting a chronic condition, like Genital Herpes, take a Cell-Salt remedy for six (6) months or up to one year. The salts are *"grouped"* or classified in the following sequence. Within each group there are specific Salts, except for Silica:

1. Calcium Salts
2. Iron Salt
3. Potassium Salts
4. Magnesium Salt
5. Sodium Salts
6. Silica

Twelve Cell-Salts: and their Respective American Numbers.

1. **Calcarea fluor (Calcium fluoride) #1**
2. Calcium phos (Calcium phosphate) #2
3. **Calcium sulph (Plaster of Paris) #3**
4. Ferrum phos (Iron phosphate) #4
5. Kali mur (Potassium chloride) #5
6. Kali phos (Potassium phosphate) #6
7. Kali sulf (Potassium sulphate) #7
8. Magnesia phos (Magnesium phosphate) #8
9. Natrum mur (Sodium chloride) #9
10. Natrum sulf (Sodium sulphate) #10
11. Natrum phos (Sodium phosphate) #11
12. Silicea (Silica) #12

Cell Salts are found throughout the blood, lymph, bones, nerves, and muscles. They play an important part in assimilating nutrients and eliminating cellular waste. Dr. Schuessler was a homeopath, so Cell-Salts are often associated with homeopathic treatment. Yet, he believed that his "biochemic system" of Cell-Salts should be separate and standalone from homeopathy. Cell-Salts are based on the body's deficiency and imbalances, not on the homeopathic principle of *"like-treats-like."* Schuessler viewed his system as more fundamental than homeopathy, but superior to it.

Bioplasma

Not sure how to treat an under-performing immune system or Genital Herpes? Start with Bioplasma. It includes all (12) twelve Cell Salts. Bioplasma is manufactured either in tablets or a sport's drink used by athletes.

Luyties Bioplasma, 500 tablet bottles in six or thirty (6x or 30x) potency.

Hylands Bioplasma http://amzn.to/2rSXUco in 500 or 1000 tablet bottles, in a standard combination of 6x and 3x potencies.

Herpes Protocol

After months dosing with Bioplasma, started Cell-Salts:

1. Kali mur, #5
2. Kali phos, #6
3. Nat mur, #9

When things calmed down, I switched to the second Cell-Salts phase:

1. Silicea, #12
2. Calc Sulph, #3

Dose and Frequency: during an active Genital Herpes outbreak, take five tablets, four times a day. Each tablet measures one grain. When two or more Cell-Salts are used, rotate them every two hours. In acute cases, a dose every half (1/2) hour may be needed, but for no more than a day or two. Thereafter, back to three or four times per day. Long-term dosing for chronic herpes infections is two or three doses daily for several months.

Put the tablets underneath the tongue and wait for them to dissolve. Do not take strong spices, stimulants like coffee, tea, tobacco, or wine within thirty (30) minutes of dosing Cell-Salt remedies. No Salts within one hour before or after meals. Taking Cell-Salts may initially aggravate detox symptoms. Headaches, slight fever, or skin issues are common. Don't get frustrated or upset. It may indicate the healing force inside your body has been stimulated. Back off if it's too intense.

Give Cell-Salts time to correct deficiencies in the immune system. Results are not as fast as traditional medicine but safer, longer lasting, and improve immune function. While treating chronic herpes, there may be an increase of outbreaks before they settle down. At such times try not to use medicated applications. They disturb the healing progress.

Aggravation occurs because the body's healing force works from inside out. It first relieves inner disorders, bringing herpes and any toxins to the surface before eliminating them. Try not to get nervous thinking that the process isn't working, or by suppressing symptoms with toxic drugs. Instead, correct eating habits and drink more water. It will assist the body's elimination pathways. You can use Cell-Salts and the homeopathic Banjari Herpes Protocol concurrently but at different times of the day.

The Hermes Protocol is a little bit like learning how to play poker. First, there are the rules to learn. Then we work within the rules to play the hands we're dealt. There are a lot of cards in a deck, as there are supplements and procedures in the Hermes Protocol. It takes time to learn their combinations and how to integrate them into a winning hand. Don't get caught bluffing. You'll lose your physical, mental, emotional, and spiritual chips.

Herpes Free may involve trying different combinations with different values for each supplement. For example, one person may find relief with five-thousand milligrams (5,000 mg) of vitamin C, while another may feel the same relief at thirty-thousand milligrams (30,000 mg). The Hermes Protocol is not a cookie cutter; it's the dough. Different ingredients comprise the taste, texture, and appearance of the body's health. Amazon.com has several cost-effective supplement options. (Ascorbic Acid Vitamin C Powder.)

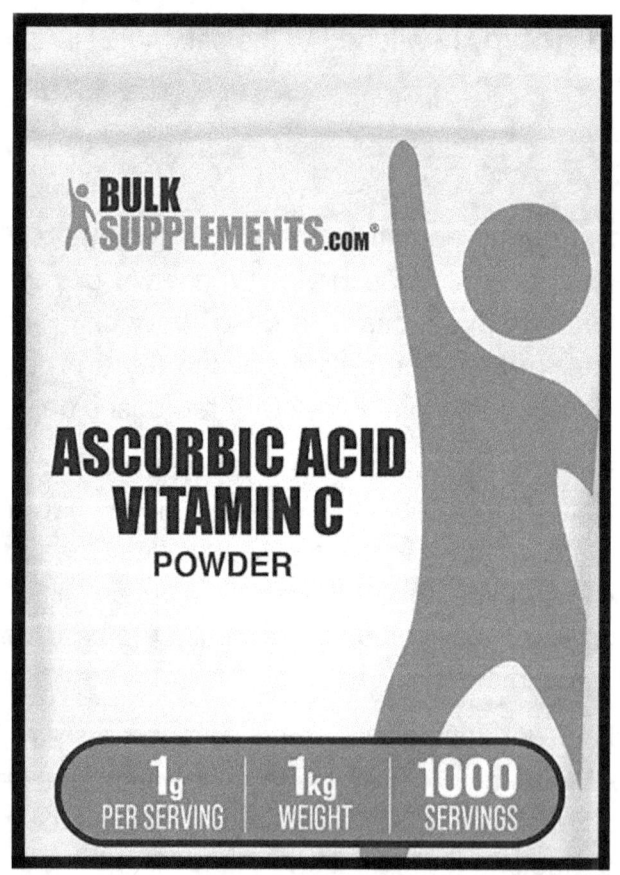

D. DMSO

April 3, 1963: discovered in 1886, DMSO (Dimethyl Sulfoxide) is an organic sulfur by-product of manufacturing paper. In 1959 scientists discovered that DMSO protected red blood cells and transplant tissue from freezing. That started the practice of preserving donor organs with DMSO. DMSO is still used for preservation of transplant organs. One of its many uses. **Stanley Jacob, MD**, as head of the University of Oregon Medical School's organ transplant team, discovered that DMSO also relieved burn pains and prevented scar tissue. When he published his findings in 1963, DMSO usage spread like wildfire. The FDA approved DMSO for the treatment for cystitis, or chronic bladder disorder.

MSM: Methylsulfonylmethane is an organic sulfur compound derived from DMSO used for joint, allergy, and gut health. MSM has many of the same properties as DMSO but is not considered as effective. But then MSM has very little controversy surrounding its use, while DMSO has been called *"the most controversial therapeutic advance of modern times."* The controversy seems more bureaucratic and economic, rather than scientific.

2017: over 29,000 DMSO indexed results showed up on pubmed.gov. It makes DMSO http://bit.ly/2Fv5IIN one of the most studied compounds of our time. Nonetheless, DMSO can't pass the required approval for other medical conditions. Yet its effectiveness and low toxicity is without question. Enough about greed and corruption, let's talk about more fundamental issues: greed, insincerity, and dishonesty.

In the real world, DMSO is used by professional athletes, from Football players to Olympic gymnasts for abnormal fluid buildup, sprains, muscle inflammation, broken bones, tennis elbow, etc., etc. Pain is reduced, swelling subsides, and function recovered.

DMSO was the first nonsteroidal anti-inflammatory discovered since aspirin. That breakthrough drove pharmaceutical companies to develop other nonsteroidal anti-inflammatories. They intuitively knew if DMSO was so effective, then other *'manufactured'* and *'marketed'* compounds could also be, but *they'll patent them*. It's the money, but the irony, *"DMSO is less toxic and has fewer side effects."* I've personally used DMSO since 2011, internally and topically for herpes, and as a 40% eye drop solution.

1975: Dr. Robert Hill, Longview, Washington, reported his eyesight studies. *"Of the 50 DMSO treated patients, 22 had improved visual acuity, nine had improved visual fields and five improved in dark adaptation. Only two patients out of the 50 continued to get worse. The remaining patients had no noticeable changes in vision. Without the treatment, it is probable that all 50 patients would have continued to regress."* http://bit.ly/2EembeI

I have used a 40% DMSO eye drop solution when my eyes felt tired or after sitting at the computer all day. There's immediate relief. After the initial stinging, the eyes feel refreshed with no pain. My vision has improved, and I seldom use my glasses anymore. The purity of

DMSO is essential. Don't buy cheap knock-off brands. Something else that is unique about DMSO: it can cross the blood brain barrier and pick up a hitchhiker. For brain related emergencies, like Herpes Encephalitis, it can be a valuable adjunct treatment option. DMSO can piggy-back an antibiotic to manage brain infections.

DMSO is also a vasodilator, which means it can increase blood flow. That's why it's popular with many athletes. It allows blood to reach football or basketball injuries that are difficult to treat. I'm confident that this book, like DMSO, will cross your brain barrier, with information to treat Genital Herpes and progress *"To-Be-Herpes-Free."*

DMSO is an effective treatment for viral infections, including herpes. In 1971, Dr. William Douglas, MD, conducted a DMSO clinical study with 46 patients infected with shingles. He applied DMSO on their lesions at various strengths, from 50% to 90%. Some were only treated with DMSO. Others combined DMSO with corticosteroid. There was no difference in the results. http://bit.ly/2DLHS5G Important to remember for future applications: "*The best results were obtained with patients treated early in the disease."*

Characteristics of DMSO

1. When DMSO is diluted with distilled water, the glass bottle gets warm. In chemistry it's called an *"exothermic reaction."* Heat is released as soon as you add water to DMSO. It's temporary, and harmless.

2. DMSO strengthens and multiplies the action of any drug dissolved in it, permitting a lower dose without reducing its effectiveness.

3. DMSO can be used as *"a penetrating carrier"* to any part of the body, passing through cellular membranes and tissues.

4. DMSO can be administered in a liquid or gel form to the skin's surface. The liquid penetrates better, but most prefer the gel. If applying DSMO to the skin, don't rub it in too hard. Just dab, apply gently, and leave it on for about 20 minutes. Then wipe off the rest.

5. The neck and face are sensitive. No higher than 50% concentration should be used.

6. Start slow, with 50% concentration until the skin builds up a tolerance. Look for any skin irritation before applying a stronger dilution.

7. IMPORTANT: The skin must be dry and clean from any contaminants.

SUMMARY: Use 99.99% pharmaceutical grade DMSO. Dilute with distilled water to lower its concentration. DMSO is an effective stand-alone **topical** treatment for Genital Herpes, or as an **internal** option to support the immune system. Topical DMSO applications for Genital Herpes outbreaks, depending on their location, can be from 50% to 90% liquid or gel strength. Liquid penetrates better; gel mixes better with other topicals. Combine colloidal silver with DMSO. Apply and leave on for about 20 minutes, then wipe off the rest. For more sensitive areas, reduce the DMSO concentration.

E. High-Dose Vitamin C

In 1936 scientists knew that Vitamin C was a powerful treatment *for herpes infections*. http://bit.ly/2FvUyhv Research showed it to be a powerful virus-killing agent.

Frederick R. Klenner, MD, (1907–1984): recorded his experience using Vitamin C for HSV- 2 in his paper, *"Clinical Guide to the Use of Vitamin C."* He was quoted, *"Some physicians would stand by and see their patient die rather than use ascorbic acid because in their finite minds it exists only as a vitamin."* http://bit.ly/2DNhqZD Dr. Klenner also emphasized that if you use Vitamin C for herpes infections it must be continued for a sufficient time. Even though cold sores seemed to heal after two Vitamin C injections, they would reoccur within 24 hours when C was discontinued.

Robert F. Cathcart, MD, (1981) also acknowledged success in treating acute herpes infections with oral Vitamin C. However, he suggested that intravenous C might be a better choice for chronic herpes infections. There's not a drug anywhere, including antivirals, which has ever *"cured"* a case of Genital Herpes. Yet, the medical community holds Vitamin C to a higher standard than their own Rx drugs.

A doctor in the *60-Minutes* documentary, *"Living Proof,"* suggested there's no "proof" that Vitamin C worked. It could just as easily have been cured by a passing bus. Passing bus? Or maybe the doctor was just passing gas.

Herpes, Shingles, and Vitamin C

Such a striking, thoughtless comment is an example of orthodox medicine's absurdity, and how it obstructs change to protect their interests. http://bit.ly/2BCTEO5 (YouTube Deleted) Wonder why?

Shingles: Frederick Klenner, MD, http://bit.ly/2DWR6iS also published his results using Vitamin C to treat eight patients with shingles. *"He gave 2,000 to 3,000 mg of Vitamin C by injection every 12 hours, supplemented by 1,000 mg in fruit juice by mouth every two hours. In seven of the eight patients treated in this manner, complete pain relief was reported within two hours of the first Vitamin C injection. All patients received a total of five to seven Vitamin C injections."*

But perhaps the most impressive results of high-dose-C for shingles was published in 1950. Researchers reported a complete resolution in 327 out of 327 shingles patients treated with intravenous Vitamin C, all within 72 hours from the start of treatment. No side effects were recorded, other than the occasional loose stools and stinky *"essential-oil-diffuser"* moments.

It's hard to ignore the facts or "studies" of Vitamin C. If you search Pub Med, there are over 50,000 studies indexed in medical literature on the extraordinary qualities of Vitamin C. So, if you ever hear there are no studies about the value of vitamin C, it's a lie. There are just no *"positive"* studies about vitamin C funded by pharmaceutical interests. Like most other natural treatments, Vitamin C is held to a different and more complex standard than conventional treatments and prescription drugs.

Studies Show:

1. Oral Vitamin C produced clear remission of symptoms in herpes labialis (cold sores). http://bit.ly/2DMURYJ

2. Vitamin C, in combination with copper, inactivated the Genital Herpes virus http://bit.ly/2nIZAXe

3. Vitamin C topical solution used against herpes lesions demonstrated significant antiviral effects. In other words, herpes went back to where it came from, and lesions healed rapidly. http://bit.ly/2EmoVHK

The Key: for effective Vitamin C therapy (orally or intravenously)

1. **QUANTITY**
2. **FREQUENCY**
3. **DURATION**

I've often heard, *"I shouldn't have to take so much Vitamin C."* That's certainly true. But for a quick recovery, it's important to use it effectively. When it comes to Genital Herpes or any disease, I'm not interested in opinions, but results. Remember, take what the body requires and wants. Not what you *think* you need or *should* take.

Forms of C

You can find Vitamin C in a variety of forms, each claiming its efficacy or bioavailability. The term bioavailability refers to the degree to which a nutrient (or drug) becomes available to the body after it has been taken. Natural and synthetic L-ascorbic acid are chemically identical, and there are no known differences in their biological activity.

Vitamin C supplements are available in many forms, there is little scientific evidence that any one form is better absorbed or more effective than another, except for Ascorbyl palmitate. (See below.) Once plasma ascorbic acid levels reach saturation, additional Vitamin C is largely excreted in urine.

1. Liposomal absorption is unlike intestinal absorption. It enters the cells directly. The fat layer of the liposome protects Vitamin C from coming in direct contact with the stomach and intestines. This prevents intestinal side effects and increases absorption from twenty percent (20%) to almost eighty percent (80%).

2. **Mineral ascorbates** are the lion's share of Vitamin C. The most common are sodium ascorbate, calcium ascorbate, and magnesium ascorbate.

3. **Sodium ascorbate** may be the safest, least expensive, high dose supplementation. Anecdotally, multi-gram doses of sodium ascorbate do not seem to adversely affect blood pressure. However, if you notice elevated blood pressures or ankle edema after high doses of sodium ascorbate, supplement with a different form of Vitamin C.

4. **Calcium ascorbate** is a popular Vitamin C supplementation, but best avoided. Excess calcium is directly correlated to increased risk of heart attacks, chronic degenerative disease, and overall *"all-cause mortality."*

5. **Magnesium ascorbate** is bioavailable and effective in reversing the damage done by excess calcium, (unless you are hypothyroid).

6. **Potassium, manganese, zinc, molybdenum, and chromium** are additional mineral ascorbates. However, they can be easily overdosed, and would avoid them.

7. **Ascorbyl Palmitate** is a fat-soluble form of Vitamin C and absorbed into the cell membrane where ascorbic acid cannot reach. It is retained in the body for a longer period. Ascorbyl palmitate is an amphipathic molecule, which means one end is water-soluble, the other fat-soluble. According to the Linus Pauling Institute, *"This dual solubility allows it to permeate the extra-cellular aqueous environment of the cell and the interior cellular environment, as well. When it is incorporated into the cell membranes of human red blood cells, ascorbyl palmitate protects them from oxidative damage and helps protect vitamin E (a fat-soluble antioxidant) from oxidation by free radicals."* Ascorbyl palmitate is an expensive way to provide multi-gram doses of ascorbate.

Options

How do you determine what the body needs? According to Dr. Levy, MD, *"Although far from perfect, one of these mechanisms, bowel tolerance, is a good starting point."* In other words, if you experience loose stools, without diarrhea, you've reached tolerance.

Dr. Robert Cathcart, MD, *"...utilizing Vitamin C in amounts just short of the dose(s) which produces diarrhea is described as... titrating to bowel tolerance. The amount of oral ascorbic acid tolerated by a patient without producing diarrhea increases somewhat proportionately to the stress or toxicity of his or her disease... lesser doses often have insignificant effect on acute symptoms but assist the body in handling the stress of disease."* http://bit.ly/2BF5KGd

Dr. Cathcart noted in his treatment of HIV/ AIDS patients bowel tolerance frequently rose to 75-100 grams per day, twenty to fifty times more than seen in healthy individuals. **Please remember that** liposome Vitamin C enjoys nearly complete absorption. It will not cause a diarrheal flush. It is considerably more bioavailable, and the following substitution schedule provides approximate values:

1,000 mg liposomal = 3,000 -- 4,000 mg powder
2,000 mg liposomal = 8,000 -- 10,000 mg powder
3,000 mg liposomal = 12,000 -- 18,000 mg powder

I do not recommend calcium ascorbate. While many people want to avoid the *"C-flush"* effect, or intestinal discomfort, every so often it's an effective way to keep the gut detoxified and clean. For those wishing to have near-complete vitamin "C" absorption, liposome-encapsulated, *"very expensive form"* of Vitamin C is optimal.

Chronic Genital Herpes Infections: if money is not a barrier, intravenous sodium ascorbate is an option. If intravenous sodium ascorbate is not available, take sodium ascorbate orally to bowel tolerance, along with a liposome form of C.

Safety, Side Effects & Myths

The safety of Vitamin C is extraordinary. There is not one case of Vitamin C toxicity anywhere in the world's medical literature. Frederick R. Klenner, MD, of North Carolina http://bit.ly/2EryXaV cured diphtheria, staph and strep infections, *herpes*, mumps, spinal meningitis, mononucleosis, shock, viral hepatitis, arthritis, and polio using high doses of Vitamin C. According to Dr. Klenner, *"Ascorbic acid is the safest and the most valuable substance available to the physician,"* and *"If you want results, use adequate ascorbic acid."* So, what do guinea pigs, fruit bats, gorilla's, lemurs, and New York City dwellers have in common? Besides being downright obnoxious at times, they cannot produce their own vitamin C.

USDA daily recommended allowance for Vitamin C is 90 mg, while all other mammals on average consume between 3,000 to 11,000 mg. per day. Since guinea pigs cannot make Vitamin C is one reason it has served science so well. *"I wonder? Guinea pigs? Humans? Who's the real guinea when it comes to scientific quackery called research?"*

Of the four mammals mentioned above, only humans have changed their dietary preferences to include meat. Yet unable to produce their own Vitamin C, gorillas, guinea pigs and fruit bats seem to know instinctually to stay healthy they must ingest enormous quantities of food containing C. You need very little Vitamin C to stay alive, but without any you die. It is called scurvy. Vitamin C is involved in making collagen, and collagen is the main protein in artery walls. No C and you literally bleed to death from the inside out. That's a margin of error of 90 mg per day to preserve your life.

At 90 mg you live. At moderate consumption of 500 to 1,500 mg you build health. You'll have fewer colds; the severity of the flu will be less. But at 8,000 to 40,000 mg per day it has therapeutic properties: antihistamine, antitoxin, antibiotic, and antiviral.

Vitamin C works like money and gasoline. Money buys effects. Even if you have a lot of it, its nature doesn't change, but its power does. And if it takes 111 gallons of gas to drive

2,789 miles from New York City to Los Angeles, you're not going to make it on 70 gallons. No matter how hard you try. Likewise, if the body wants 40,000 mg of Vitamin C to fight a herpes infection, 6,000 mg won't do. The key to Vitamin C supplementation is to take enough, often enough, and long enough.

A word of caution for those with kidney disease or compromised renal function. It is essential you work with a qualified health practitioner before dosing with Vitamin C.

Also, if you've been taking calcium supplements for years, without extra vitamin K-2, it's possible that extensive calcium deposits have accumulated throughout the body, including your arteries. Vitamin C dissolves calcium, so when you start taking C for the first time, greater amounts of calcium will be dissolved. Stay well hydrated, start with smaller doses of Vitamin C, and increase the dosage slowly over time.

For those seeking objective measurements, get a *periodic urinary calcium measurement test* from your doctor. It indicates the amount of calcium being excreted from the body. Once that's stabilized, then increase the Vitamin C amount. Also, if you have ANY medical condition that needs to be treated and monitored, always check with your health care provider before taking larger doses of C or any vitamin.

Ascorbic Acid is the straight form of Vitamin C and not buffered. It can aggravate the stomach, especially for those with GI issues, GERD, or ulcers. A buffered form of Vitamin C, like Sodium Ascorbate is ideal for mega-dosing.

WARNING: large doses of Vitamin C are contraindicated with certain blood diseases including **sickle-cell anemia, hemochromatosis, and thalassemia.** Keep the following considerations in mind:

1. **Vitamin C increases** iron and decreases copper absorption.

2. **Ascorbic Acid,** the acid form of Vitamin C, may aggravate stomach ulcers.

3. **Ascorbic Acid** can cause diarrhea, which may NOT be a desired outcome.

4. **A myth** that is often bantered about as truth is that large doses of Vitamin C trigger kidney stones. To date it has never been proven, documented, or substantiated, but is often quoted by critics of Vitamin C. The evidence indicates this claim is false.

5. **There are a few other myths,** but my favorite is that Vitamin C increases the risk of cancer. The irony, the latest cancer research shows just the opposite http://bit.ly/2GxjOVV.

F. Low Dose Naltrexone (LDN)

Forty years ago, two researchers from Penn State University, Drs. Ian Zagon and Pat McLaughlin, discovered that Low Dose Naltrexone (**LDN**) helped relieve symptoms of multiple sclerosis (MS). Since then, they've studied the effects of **LDN** on a wide range of diseases. They isolated LDN's key endorphin responsible for its healing effects. They named it OGF (Opioid Growth Factor). They've successfully treated patients with difficult pancreatic and liver cancers. To date, more than 70 studies and reports have been published about LDN. And as of 2023 it's estimated that more than 350,000 patients worldwide are benefiting from LDN. This author is one of them.

Naltrexone is FDA approved: to treat heroin addiction for over 20 years. They use it in a 50-mg dose to *"block"* opioid receptors, so addicts can no longer get *"high."* From this idea, Drs. Zagon & McLaughlin created *"Low-Dose-Naltrexone"* in a small three-to-four-and-a-half (3-to-4.5) mg dose. Research found it to be beneficial for autoimmune conditions such as lupus, rheumatoid arthritis, multiple sclerosis, and cancer, as well as infectious diseases such as HIV and Genital Herpes. http://bit.ly/2DMpOs0

LDN at bedtime boosts the immune system by stimulating the body's own natural defenses. Research studies indicate that endorphin secretions play a key role in modulating the immune system. If LDN is taken at bedtime, it blocks certain opioid receptors during the early morning hours (from 2 AM to 4 AM). Afterwards, it induces a prolonged up-regulation of the immune system. In plain immune armed forces dialogue, *"More good guys come out to fight the bad guys."*

Considering the impact of LDN http://bit.ly/2EoosVO on the immune system (2008 YouTube Video), Genital Herpes may be influenced by LDN therapy. Talk to your *"alternative"* doctor or go to www.LDNscience.org to find one and learn more about the therapeutic benefits of LDN. It's *"the most credible up-to-date information website about Low Dose Naltrexone (LDN) for Physicians, Researchers, and Patients."*

Most traditional physicians or providers will not prescribe LDN, unless you're a heroin addict. Otherwise, they may look at you with that pedigree *"I'm the Doctor"* haughtiness and wonder aloud if you shouldn't be on *'some kind of antidepressant.'*

G. Chlorine Dioxide or MMS1

All YouTube MMS Videos are Unavailable. ACCOUNTS have been Terminated. Why?

MMS + 4% Hydrochloric Acid = Chlorine Dioxide

MMS + 4% HCl (Hydrochloric Acid) = MMS1 or Chlorine Dioxide (CD)

The above formula is how to make Chlorine Dioxide, or what Jim Humble refers to as MMS1. However, Master Mineral Solution or MMS are the terms most people use when talking about Chlorine Dioxide, even though technically it's not correct. The acronym MMS is un-activated 22.4% Sodium Chlorite solution ($NaClO_2$) in water. Not Chlorine Dioxide, which is MMS1. Don't worry, it gets worse. Just kidding. I thought I'd try to clean up the mess before getting started. The terminology of MMS is the most confusing and difficult part of the protocol.

Chlorine Dioxide and MMS1: are interchangeable terms for activated MMS. (See table below) Take your time reading this condensed explanation of MMS. It's a simple subject muddied by acronyms, chemistry, and terminology, making it more confusing than it is. Absorb as much as you can, and then take advantage of the many internet blogs to learn more. If you can't recall formulas, MMS names, solutions, or acronyms, refer to this book for an abbreviated explanation.

1. **Sodium Chlorite** = Un-activated MMS or Master Mineral Solution
2. **Un-activated MMS** = 22.4% solution of Sodium Chlorite ($NaClO_2$)
3. **Activated MMS** = MMS1 or Chlorine Dioxide
4. **Chlorine Dioxide** = MMS1 and is often referred to as *"activated"* MMS

Introduction

Most readers will not be familiar with the terms Sodium Chlorite or Chlorine Dioxide (CD) but may have heard the acronyms MMS or Master Mineral Solution. It's the label Jim Humble attached to un-activated MMS. He thought it was *"miraculous"* that MMS saved the life of his friend dying from malaria.

Remember, Chlorine Dioxide and MMS1 are the same solutions. One is the technical term, the other a popularized version coined by Jim Humble. The internet is bursting with MMS testimonials from every part of the globe. Many in writing, more in video format. But there are also many *"quack-monials"* from those who have a vested-interest in seeing MMS fear-mongered. Hoping people will become too confused and afraid to use it. Their favorite smear-tactic is: *"Would you drink bleach?"* Of course not, who would be that Wikipedia? But then Chlorine Dioxide is not chlorine. Like sodium chloride is not Sodium Chlorite. One is table salt. Which one? With the letter "d."

Trying to discredit MMS by saying it's *"bleach,"* is like saying water buffalo come from chickens. Yes, both are animals, made up of living cells, and use energy. But they come from different genetic planets. Earth to Mars.

MMS1/Chlorine Dioxide (ClO2) and table salt (NaCl): both have the chlorine element in their composition. The "Cl" stands for chlorine. But chlorine is not dangerous. Unless you consider table salt poison. Yet the FDA and medical establishment keep slandering, criticizing MMS with simple minded scare tactics that don't hold up to sixth grade chemistry. Household bleach, which is sodium hypochlorite (NaClO), also has Cl in its formula. But the chlorine (Cl) is in a different form, and in some cases can be unsafe. Yet bleach is not labeled with a skull and crossbones poison symbol. Like many products, it has warnings. They're usually exaggerated for litigation purposes. For example, it states that Clorox bleach, *"Causes irreversible eye damage and skin burns."*

By now I should be blind and look like Edward Scissorhands from doing laundry. The only thing I've ever felt is smarmy. Not even skin burns. They use the word *"industrial"* bleach because it makes it sound more hazardous. But think about it, most things are made in factories, it's an industry. There's nothing inherently dangerous about being industrial. It's manufactured marketing.

I don't splash chlorine, after shave, or alcohol in my eyes. It would sting, irritate, and even cause some damage. But after an all-day computer marathon, my eyes are fatigued. That's when I use a forty percent (40%) DMSO eye drop solution to bring them back to life. I've used a MMS1 solution but prefer DMSO for its dilation effect. After the initial sting, my eyes always feel better. How industrial. Also, if Chlorine Dioxide (CD) is so toxic, why is it used in so many municipal water districts as a disinfectant? It's the safest and most effective purifier, and at low concentration, it barely reacts with organic matter and forms few by-products.

When two sides are polarized about the good, bad, and half-truths, look at motivation, science, and its source. Not the fiction. The best advice I can give is what the farmer said to the stranded city slicker. *"Let's make chicken salad out of this chicken sheet situation."* We must be willing to take the time to learn the facts and truth about MMS and DMSO, and not take vested interests propaganda at face value.

MMS misinformation is all over the internet. It makes it difficult to separate truth from fiction unless you're a chemist. The worst offender is Wikipedia. Using misleading and deceptive transcripts, it borders on juvenile fiction about Jim Humble and MMS. But maybe the biggest threat to MMS is not Wiki, Pharma, FDA, or CNN, but our own fear and apathy. It takes time and effort to learn something new. Then courage to act on it. Congratulations for being brave.

Parallels to Marijuana

The use and history of marijuana is like that of Chlorine Dioxide or MMS1. In 2015, a US Marine Corps veteran returned from overseas with post-traumatic stress disorder (PTSD). As of this writing, he is facing possible life imprisonment for treating his condition with marijuana. According to his wife, before he started using marijuana to ease his PTSD. *"He was taking thirteen (13) pills a day, and it was killing his liver. He was having all these issues with his body and wanted to try something more natural to see if he could do without so many pills a day."*

It's way past medieval and draconian midnight for change. Although many states have passed legislation allowing marijuana for medical and/or recreational use, more need to follow. When it happens, crime rates drop, tax revenues increase, and there is less pain for returning PTSD veterans. Yet there are still those who continue to dole out harsh punishment for soldiers or patients in chronic pain who dare to use marijuana.

The same was true for Daniel Smith, who faced life imprisonment for selling MMS to people in need. U.S. Department of Justice website: *"Seller of Miracle Mineral Solution Convicted for Marketing Toxic Chemical as a Miracle Cure."* It's time to assert that in the twenty (20) years since Jim Humble's re-discovery of MMS, not one person has died from using it. I wonder why they are still letting us take aspirins. The link below is from May 28, 2015, Department of Justice: Seller of *"Miracle Mineral Solution"* Convicted for Marketing Toxic Chemical as a Miracle Cure. http://bit.ly/2DKKalG

September 2018 Update: Daniel Smith is home; although, still in custody in his apartment. The Bureau of Prisons (BOP) still controlled his every move. He had to give notice to request leaving his apartment, for a job interview, going to church, shopping, or having someone visit. This custodial monitoring lasted four and a half (4 1/2) months, and then he reported to his Parole Officer for an additional four years.

Changing our beliefs is difficult. Most important discoveries are first rejected, ridiculed, and opposed. And if all else fails, the people responsible are prosecuted and jailed. By the time we hear about it on Fake News Networks, it's been massaged and manipulated to enhance those special sponsorships and interests that will benefit most. The most famous recent example was Drs. Barry Marshall and Robin Warren of Australia. They discovered that *h-pylori* caused ulcers, and not stress. And as a result, both were ridiculed and hounded for a quarter century. At the time, conventional thinking was no bacterium could live in the acid environment of the human stomach. Fast forward to 2005, when they were both awarded the Nobel Prize in medicine for their discovery!

MMS in *alternative* therapy. Do your research. That's what I did before putting a drop of MMS1 into my body. I don't recommend following any advice or treatment blindly, including mine from this book, your doctors, or any unconventional protocols. Verify the information via footnotes, links, and through reliable organizations. In some ways, that's what you're doing right now by reading this book. Also check out www.JimHumbleBooks.co

When you think about it, *"My Friend, The Enemy"* is nothing more than a personal accounting and *research* about my experience into being Genital Herpes Free. Maybe the words in this book will help you decide whether to research or use MMS for your chronic Genital Herpes infections.

Chlorine Dioxide (CD): purifies water, sanitizes hospital floors, decontaminates slaughterhouses, and disinfects vegetables. Compare *"zero"* deaths, to millions caused by pharmaceutical drugs. In one year in the U.S. alone, more than 15,000 die from taking Ibuprofen and Aspirin. It's insanity that CD is even an issue. The only other time I've seen such an uproar is when alternative medicine tries to shed light on the shadowy underbelly of vaccines. *"A group of researchers meticulously reviewed the statistical evidence, and their findings are absolutely shocking. It presents compelling evidence that today's (medical) system frequently causes more harm than good."* Life Extension 2004 http://bit.ly/2nqNk7b

MMS Chemistry and How to Make MMS1:

1. **Start** with Sodium Chlorite (un-activated MMS). Do not ingest.
2. **Activate** Sodium Chlorite (MMS) with 4% HCl, hydrochloric acid.
3. **Wait** about 90 seconds. It turns into Chlorine Dioxide, or MMS1.
4. **Chlorine Dioxide** (CD) is the technical term for MMS1.

Two *other forms* of activated MMS:

1. **CDS** (Chlorine Dioxide solution)
2. **CDH** (Chlorine Dioxide holding).

Both are a form of Chlorine Dioxide, but they function in diverse ways, depending on an individual's sensitivity and goals. I've used all three in treating a variety of health issues. Please do your research once you are familiar with the standard MMS/CD protocols.

Current Products

You may have used Chlorine Dioxide and not known it. The following products contain Chlorine Dioxide approved by the Food and Drug Administration (FDA). They are manufactured by Frontier Pharmaceutical, Alcide, Bioxy, and others for skin and oral care:

1. Cankers Away
2. DioxiRinse™ Mouthwash
3. DioxiBrite™ Toothpaste
4. DioxiWhite™ Pro Teeth Whitener

5. WhiteLasting™ Maintenance Gel
6. BioClenz™ Dental Unit Waterline Cleaner
7. Penetrator™ Periodontal Gel
8. Simply Clear™ Acne Treatment

History

Sodium Chlorite (un-activated MMS) has been used in alternative medicine for more than seventy (70) years to prevent colds and treat a variety of microbial conditions. Jim Humble *"re-discovered"* that if you *"activate"* Sodium Chlorite with an acid it turns into Chlorine Dioxide, or what today is called MMS1, a *"more effective agent"* than Sodium Chlorite. *One more time.* You make Chlorine Dioxide (MMS1) by activating Sodium Chlorite (MMS) with a four percent (4%) solution of hydrochloric acid.

While prospecting for minerals in the jungles of South America, Jim Humble's colleague was infected with a deadly form of malaria, which often killed its victims within hours without medical intervention. In a final effort to bring about some relief, Jim treated his friend with water purification drops. A solution of Sodium Chlorite that Jim used to make suspect water potable. To everyone's amazement, the stricken man recovered. Upon returning to the States, Jim was determined to find out how and why. Over the next few years, he fined-tuned his MMS protocol and then went to Africa to verify his findings against malaria. Jim personally treated thousands of malaria victims and another 75,000 people through missionaries.

Jim Humble began his career as a research engineer in the aerospace industry. He speaks of his career rarely, but rumor has it that he worked on lunar vehicles, intercontinental missiles, atomic bombs, and the first vacuum tune computer. The consummate inventor. In fact, it's said he invented the first automatic garage door! Many thanks from all of us who live in the snow.

He's said many times, *"My most important discovery yet has been how to eradicate the dreaded malaria parasite from the lives of many who are currently suffering this beastly condition."* Jim has not benefited from the sale of MMS. He divested his interest from making money when he realized financial gain could be construed as a conflict of interest. Instead, he concentrated his efforts on getting the word out, before money-interests and regulatory bodies tried to shut down MMS for good. Because of the FDA crackdown, Jim Humble organized his protocols under a religious *"sacrament"* umbrella in 2010, *The Genesis II Church of Health and Healing*.

As of August 2017: there are 214 "Church-Chapters" in 135 countries, with 2,836 members, 1,841 Health Ministers, and 101 Bishops. There are over one-million views (1,000,000) on the *"MMS Testimonials"* YouTube channel: including 75,000 weekly for the

G2Voice Broadcast. Millions have used and benefited from MMS1 worldwide. There was a YouTube video of the history of the Genesis II Church, but *"This video is no longer available because the YouTube account associated with this video has been terminated."* http://bit.ly/2Gsx91E (Account Terminated)

Mode of Kill Action

Jim Humble is a great humanitarian. There is no doubt about that. He also must have been a dependable NASA engineer. However, at times his understanding of chemistry and body biochemistry is incomplete, which he's admitted. The most common errors are that human body cells repel Chlorine Dioxide (CD), and that it can differentiate between good and bad bacteria. In his books Jim mentions that CD *"somehow"* works differently on different pathogens. That's not true, but there are those who believe his opinions.

Chlorine Dioxide (MMS1) kills bacteria in low concentration through protein synthesis disruption and enzyme inactivation. Similar to the non-toxic mechanism of common antibiotics. However, in high doses it can hurt body tissue, as well as that of pathogens. Since MMS1 acts both on good and unhealthy bacteria, taking probiotics is recommended after internal MMS1 treatments.

Jim Humble's harmless claim was a bit naive. Just because you don't see it doesn't mean it's not there or causing harm. I've taken large doses of pure Chlorine Dioxide and inhaled full breaths of it. It's in *"the dose that makes the poison"* is a basic principle of toxicology. MMS1 doses should be kept reasonable. The good thing about Chlorine Dioxide it works in low doses, compared to antibiotics and other disinfectants.

Jim was wrong about MMS1 lasting only an hour in our bodies. Rats are not human, but studies showed Sodium Chlorite reached peak blood levels in eight (8) hours, and twenty-one percent (21%) was still there after 72 hours. Medicating every hour with large doses may not be a promising idea unless you have a disease like malaria and are fighting for your life. Extra precautions must be employed in people with *glucose-6-phosphate-dehydrogenase* deficiency disease. They are sensitive to oxidants of all kinds.

Chlorine Dioxide is a free radical, so antioxidants quench it back into a chlorite form. Do not consume antioxidant supplements, natural juices, or rich antioxidant foods while taking MMS. Lemon or lime juice has vitamin C, so they're not a good mix. Other antioxidants to avoid include vitamins E, A, CoQ10, flavonoids, Beta-carotene, Lycopene, and Lutein.

A Word of Caution: do not make Sodium Chlorite on your own. Buy it and the four-percent (4%) Hydrochloric Acid activator from a reputable company and approved *"water purification"* vendors http://www.wpsuppliers.com. I've never ingested MMS2 or calcium hypochlorite. It's the second protocol Jim Humble talks about in his books. Swallowing too many capsules containing solid calcium hypochlorite could *"burn"* the stomach lining. It reacts with gastrointestinal acid to produce chlorine gas. But instead of just making the public aware, like drinking too much whiskey, Big Pharma tried to degrade the entire Chlorine Dioxide process.

Dosage

Large doses of MMS1 may cause nausea, vomiting or diarrhea. That's probably not a Herxheimer reaction, but the body's attempt to rid itself of MMS1. I've not experienced those symptoms, but others have. To be fair, Jim Humble is constantly addressing the issue of taking too much MMS1. He stresses backing off if there is too much discomfort. One thing that may help is taking a dose per pound of a person's weight, rather than simply counting the number of drops. Criticism and critique do not negate the usefulness of MMS1. Staying within the "No-Adverse-Effect-Levels," MMS1 is extremely safe and practical. I'd take MMS1 any day before antibiotics. Even at damaging levels.

There is a significant benefit from taking low dose MMS1. It stimulates white blood cells to produce cytokines, which in turn stimulate other white blood cells, thereby activating the immune system. Another MMS1 benefit is that it destroys most venom and poisons. Compared to anti-venoms that cost tens of $1,000, have a short shelf life, and hospitals seldom stock, it may be wise for that reason to keep some MMS and an activator handy.

Starting Protocol

Jim Humble over time adjusted his starting protocol. He understood and responded to criticism that not everyone is critically ill with malaria. Today he suggests starting out at one-fourth of a drop (1/4) of MMS1. The *"new"* three golden rules of dosing are a one-fourth (1/4) drop every hour:

1. **If you are getting better**, don't change anything.
2. **If you are feeling worse**, cut your next dose in half.
3. **Not feeling worse or better** (nothing has changed) increase the dose.

Warning!

Keep MMS out of the reach of children and pets, and DO NOT keep it in unmarked bottles or glass. MMS has no smell and is almost impossible to tell apart from water. Some have drunk as much as half (1/2) a glass of MMS before realizing they were not drinking water. If you drink too much MMS, either by mistake or on purpose, immediately drink as much water with salt as possible. Try to induce vomiting. Use one (1) tablespoon of salt per one liter/quart of water. Then drink more and try to vomit again. Do this several times. If you still feel bad, go to the hospital.

Before using MMS as outlined in this book for Genital Herpes, read Jim Humble's book, *MMS Health Recovery Guidebook,* at www.mmsnews.is (Link Broken or Site Can't be Reached??)

Topical & Internal

Topical MMS for Genital Herpes

1. **Four (4) drops** of un-activated MMS in a small dish,
2. **Add four (4) drops** of 4% HCL,
3. **Wait 30 to 60 seconds** (it's now activated or MMS1),
4. **Add four (4) drops** of DMSO to the solution,
5. **Wait two (2) minutes and mix in six (6) drops** of distilled water, and
6. **When ready,** use a Q-Tip, lightly apply the mixture to your blisters.

Starting Procedure: Protocol 1000 and Genital Herpes (Internal)

1st day: every hour take one-quarter drop (1/4) of activated MMS (MMS1) for eight (8) hours. Mix a one-drop (1) solution, then add four (4) ounces of distilled water. Pour off one (1) ounce and drink that. Discard the remaining three (3) ounces down the drain. Make a new batch every hour and consume within sixty-seconds (60) after MMS is activated. *(Detailed activation instruction below.)*

2nd and 3rd days: one-half (1/2) drop of MMS1 every one-hour for eight (8) hours. Follow the same procedure as above, only this time pour off two-ounces (2), drink that, and discard the remaining two-ounces.

4th day: three-quarter drop of MMS1 every one-hour for eight (8) hours. Follow the same procedure as above but this time drink three (3) ounces, discarding one (1) ounce. That's the starting process before advancing to Protocol 1000.

Protocol 1000

From a one-half (1/2) drop to three (3) drops per hour, until the lesions are healed. If I felt a hint of lightheadedness or nausea, I adjusted my dosage down, but did not stop taking the drops. I avoided taking Vitamin C or other antioxidants. No coffee, tea, milk, or alcohol—with one exception. I had my morning cup of coffee but gave myself a two-hour window before starting the protocol. If I had a busy schedule, I'd prepare the solution for the day in a one liter/quart bottle. Watch Jim Humble on YouTube http://bit.ly/2GrP6gW explain the various MMS Protocols. **(All MMS Videos Unavailable, YouTube Accounts Terminated since 1st Edition 2018!!)**

Step One: Protocol 1000

1. **Always** use an empty, clean, dry, four-ounce (4) glass.

2. **Tilt** the glass or put a chip under one side. Drip the MMS drops into the lower side of the glass. Hold the eye dropper straight up and down when releasing drops.

3. **Using a four-percent** (4%) solution of HCl, add the same amount of activator drops on top of the MMS drops. For example, if you used four (4) drops of MMS, add four drops of four-percent (4%) HCl.

Step Two:

Swirl the drops a little as you wait about sixty (60) seconds. The mixture should turn amber and let off gas. Try not to inhale the MMS1 gas.

Step Three: Dr. Andreas Kalcker, Straight Talk on MMS http://bit.ly/2FvO1U9 (YouTube Account Terminated)

1. **After the mixture** turns amber, add four (4) ounces/120 ml of clean drinking water.

2. **Purified water** is OK, distilled better. If the taste of MMS1 is objectionable, some juices are fine if they don't contain harmful preservatives and/or added Vitamin C. These cancel out the effectiveness of MMS1.

3. **Never use tap water.** Some bottled water contains fluoride, chlorine, and other harmful substances. Distilled water is a better choice.

4. **If you are taking** one (1) drop of MMS1, pour off three (3) ounces of water and drink one (1) ounce.

5. **Drink the dose fresh**, in less than one (1) minute.

Some people find the taste of MMS1 difficult to swallow. Pathogens in the body create an aversion to whatever threatens them as a survival mechanism. Keep a positive attitude and do the best you can. Personally, I find this Rx dictatorial censorship more difficult to swallow. Historically, I've seen it in Germany, Russia, Cuba, and many South American Countries. It does not bode well for the U.S. and our Democracy. Pharmaceutical money. Not our health and well-being.

H. Proteolytic Enzymes

Whether breaking down food, the cell walls of a virus, rebuilding an injury, or quenching inflammation, enzymes are catalysts and play a key role in human biological processes and the life cycle of many pathogens.

Enzymes fall into three categories:
1. Food enzymes,
2. Digestive enzymes, and
3. Proteolytic or Systemic enzymes

Food enzymes: are found in raw food. To increase their intake, eat a healthy organic diet, rich in vegetables. Avoid processed foods. They're dead. Cooking destroys most food enzymes. It's best to lightly steam veggies.

Digestive enzymes: describe their purpose. They help break down fiber, protein, carbohydrates, and fats. Many people require fewer gastrointestinal medications when they supplement with digestive enzymes and *"Betaine HCl"* with Pepsin.

Proteolytic or Systemic enzymes: help build, maintain overall health, clean the blood, and *address specific health issues such as:*

1. Control inflammation throughout the body.
2. Repair the cardiovascular system.
3. Improve blood flow.
4. Prevent or dissolve blood clots.
5. Dissolve plaque in arteries.
6. Optimize the immune system.
7. Help alleviate the effects of allergies.
8. Improve exercise recovery times.

These benefits stem from proteolytic enzymes ability to break down undesirable proteins in the bloodstream and soft tissue. They are potent virus fighters and an excellent therapy for Genital Herpes, to digest the protective protein layer that surrounds the virus. Eliminating herpes coating leaves it unprotected and vulnerable to the immune system.

1995, Dr. Billigmann published a study with enzyme therapy in the treatment of Herpes Zoster, or shingles. The enzyme preparation showed identical effectiveness as the drug Acyclovir. It confirmed the results of a prior study. *"Enzymes have few side-effects and provide significant pain relief for the patient (Bartsch 1974; Scheef 1987)."*

In a perfect world, we would all eat organic, unprocessed foods, naturally high in active enzymes. From Columbine and Genital Herpes, we know this world is not perfect. Too often we eat food that is enzyme deficient. The body compensates. It's forced to stop producing proteolytic enzymes and instead produces pancreatic enzymes to break down the dead food we eat.

Additional Proteolytic Benefits: http://bit.ly/2BDISGY

1. Reduces systemic inflammation for cancer, fibromyalgia, fatigue.
2. Breaks down and removes circulating immune complexes (CICs).
3. Dissolves fibrin, leading to the breakup of arterial plaque.
4. Helps avoid the risk of DVT (Deep Vein Thrombosis).
5. Boosts the immune system, improves body alkalinity.
6. Kills bacteria, viruses, and other invading pathogens.
7. Helps with autoimmune diseases.
8. Reduces the risk and response to food and pollen allergies.
9. Accelerates recovery from sprains, fractures, bruises, contusions.
10. Supports multiple sclerosis.
11. Eliminates plaque from teeth.
12. Improves sinusitis and asthma.
13. Dissolves arterial scar tissue.
14. Aids in cleansing and detoxification.

The regular use of proteolytic enzymes can be an invaluable addition to a daily Genital Herpes and immune health regimen. Herpes is a protein/amino acid-based virus. Proteolytic enzymes between meals go into the bloodstream and digest these invaders. Proteolytic enzymes should be in vegetarian capsules that can resist the low ph of the stomach and pass into the small intestine to do their healing work. http://bit.ly/2nr4SQv

Give proteolytic enzymes a helping hand:

1. Add more raw foods to your diet,
2. Cut out all highly processed foods,
3. Cut down on over-cooked foods, and
4. Chew food thoroughly so it mixes with the enzymes in saliva.

Herpes does not need to be active to experience the benefits of systemic enzymes. They help absorb vital nutrients from the foods we eat, thereby promoting better health.

Dosage: The first couple of weeks take one capsule a day, at least one-hour before eating. Taking them first thing in the morning on an empty with a large glass of water is an excellent option.

1. Then increase the dosage to two capsules a day.
2. If there is no discomfort, increase to three capsules.
3. One-to-three capsules a day is the optimum long-term dose.

Safety and Side Effects: do not take proteolytic enzymes if nursing or pregnant, have a history of ulcers, or taking blood thinners. Do NOT take them at least a week before having elective surgery. If in doubt, contact your health care provider and make certain proteolytic enzymes are appropriate for your health condition.

Can you take too many, too often? Absolutely! Proteolytic enzymes work as a natural blood thinner. If the dosage is higher than the body can handle, it will increase the tendency to have spontaneous nosebleeds or increased rectal bleeding with hemorrhoids. If you experience any intestinal discomfort, back down or stop until symptoms subside.

Chapter 11: Supplements

Do you have a lobby? I don't, but then I live in a modest townhome. However, if you ever get a chance to visit a pharmaceutical company, they have gigantic lobbies in CNN, the New York Times, college universities, scientific journals, and our watchdog, the FDA. It's the *"Anti-Supplement Lobby."*

Aug 23, 2017: CNN Health posted the following piece of propaganda. *"High doses of vitamin B6 & B12 tied to lung cancer risk, study says."* http://cnn.it/2Ftih1J Like when the tobacco industry "swore" nicotine was not addictive. The Advisory Board of the Orthomolecular Medicine News Service (OMNS) was more direct, *"It's a crock."* http://orthomolecular.org/

Click on their website if *"you've had enough of vitamin-bashing newspaper, magazine and TV reports."* Sign up for the truth about vitamins. In their Jan 2017 edition, there's an article on the safety of supplements http://bit.ly/2GuC42k *"No Deaths from Supplements."*

Dr. Andrew Saul, Editor-in-Chief, *"Hospitals are the real problem. They are the third leading cause of death in America. That dietary supplements kill no one is completely ignored."* Who would pay their salaries? Please do not to be fooled by anti-supplement articles. Remember, the media is on alert for *"fake scare stories."* That way we'll impassively, yet fearfully, sit through all their manufactured commercials and buy the stuff we don't need. Modern medicine knows how to diagnose and treat **"disease-symptoms"** with drugs and surgery. They know next to squat about supplements. But they want them stopped because they interfere with drug treatments. **Translation:** you may no longer need drugs if you take the right supplements.

You've heard or seen football fans at tailgate parties yell. *"Quod ali cibus est Hamburger, aliis fuat acre Hotdog venenum."* What is Hamburger for one man, is a poisonous Hotdog to another. In barbecue jargon, *"One man's meat is another man's poison."* The author takes complete credit for exploiting football fans, Latin, and the English language all in one sentence. Thank you, Officer Brezhnev. Remember, stay mindful when taking any kind of medicine or supplement. Risk-free to one-man, poisonous snake to the next.

A. Immune Support Vitamins

Boost Your Immune System with proper nutrition and supplements to reduce the frequency and duration of Genital Herpes outbreaks. Part of that insurance is to make sure the body has an adequate intake of:

1. Vitamin A
2. Zinc
3. Selenium
4. Vitamin E
5. Vitamin C
6. Multiple Vitamin/Mineral Supplement

Low Arginine Diet: proper stress management, absorbing adequate amounts of vitamins and minerals. Then we look at specific supplements that may directly impact our immune system. Like all props to healing, the goal is for our immune system to keep herpes dormant. Because of individual differences, the difficulty is discovering an effective combination. That's why we do a Hair Tissue Mineral Analysis (HTMA).

The following five (5) vitamins are a good foundation. Dosage recommendations are for adults only and will be explained in detail in the next section. Take the following dosage during an active Genital Herpes outbreak:

1. Vitamin A: during an active outbreak take 25,000 to 50,000 IU daily for seven (7) days, then reduce the dosage to 15,000 IU for seven more. After that, take 10,000 IU daily. Use natural vitamin A only.

2. Vitamin C: take 10,000 mg, or an amount equal to bowel tolerance, in divided doses. The upper limit will be different for each person. Then back off until stools are soft, but not runny. Consider taking this amount until the infection has almost healed..

3. Vitamin E: up to 400 IU per day with mixed tocopherols and tocotrienols.

4. Zinc: take 25 mg two times a day during an outbreak and recovery state. Thereafter, depending on copper status, take 15 to 25 mg per day for maintenance. A word of caution regarding zinc and copper. They are antagonists and decrease or block the absorption of the other. Supplement them at different times or days. The HTMA analysis is the best way to monitor zinc and copper levels.

5. Selenium: up to 200 mcg per day.

(1) Vitamin A

Vitamin A Deficiency: increases the risk for many viral illnesses, including Genital Herpes. An important fat-soluble vitamin, it's found in fatty foods and best taken with those same foods. Vitamin A is required to preserve our eyesight. It strengthens the skin and regulates cell growth and hormone synthesis. The brain uses it to process information. It's found in every cell of the body for respiration and energy production. If the body is low in vitamin A, our energy levels suffer. Infections and cancer can develop. According to the World Health Organization, *"Vitamin A deficiency is the leading cause of preventable blindness in children and increases the risk of disease and death from severe infections."* http://bit.ly/2rRz7FM

Vitamin A deficiency can cause night blindness, or trouble seeing in the dark, and increases the risk for cardiovascular disease, macular degeneration, cataracts, osteoporosis, diarrheal diseases, and many other viral illnesses. After 1940 and more than thirty (30) clinical trials, vitamin A was commonly referred to as the anti-infective vitamin. It plays a key role in healing herpes infections and is a crucial factor in skin and mucous membrane integrity. http://bit.ly/2EpcafF

A 2000 University of Washington clinical study showed a moderate deficiency in vitamin A created a significant risk in women developing Genital Herpes infections. While the study did not state vitamin A prevents herpes, it implied that "A" plays a key role in supporting a healthy immune system. Healthy immune system, fewer herpes outbreaks. http://bit.ly/2DMJdci

Safety and Side Effects: take a pre-formed vitamin A, not beta-carotene. Many have trouble converting carotenes to the active form of vitamin A. Those with kidney, liver issues, or high blood pressure, consult with your health care provider before taking vitamin A, or any supplement.

(2) Vitamin C

During an active Genital Herpes outbreak, keep the body saturated with vitamin C, supplementing every two-to-three (2-3) hours to bowel tolerance, or until symptoms subside. To monitor your levels, Vitamin C Test Strips are available at Amazon.

Vitamin C is critical in maintaining proper immune function:

1. Strengthens white blood cells, boosts interferon levels.
2. Free radical scavenger, protects tissues from oxidative stress.
3. Effects all body processes, diseases, and syndromes.
4. Acts as an electron donor for at least eight enzymes.
5. Inhibits viral infectivity by affecting viral replication.
6. Antioxidant that helps alleviate oxidative stress, and inflammation.

"Don't leave home without your C"

If using Vitamin C to recover from a genital or oral herpes infection, use it effectively. As always, the three keys to using Vitamin C are:

1. **QUANTITY:** how much.
2. **FREQUENCY:** how often.
3. **DURATION:** for how long.

A repeated *word of caution* for those with *kidney disease* that have not progressed to a state of acute or chronic renal failure: Keep well hydrated and make sure never to take **calcium ascorbate**. Drink two quarts of "purified" water daily and work with a qualified health practitioner.

(3) Vitamin E

Clinical Studies: showed strong support for the use of vitamin E for herpes infections. Vitamin E is also neuro-protective and can help relieve nerve pain during outbreaks. A study published June 2006 in *Alternative Medicine Review* expressed concern about the safety and efficacy of Acyclovir, the most prescribed pharmaceutical antiviral drug for Genital Herpes. It suggested that dietary modifications along with natural dietary supplements, including oral and topical vitamin E, might be more beneficial. View natural remedies http://bit.ly/2GuRF1K for Herpes Simplex. An earlier study in 1997, *Antiviral Research*, compared vitamin E to Acyclovir in guinea pigs. The results showed that Acyclovir was effective in killing the herpes virus, but vitamin E did a notably better job healing skin lesions. http://bit.ly/2DLo9Tv

Vitamin E Deficiency: symptoms may include anemia, kidney disease, cystic fibrosis, fatigue, impaired circulation, general poor health, poor muscle development or muscle wasting, and asthma. Take up to 400 IU per day of natural vitamin E with mixed tocopherols and tocotrienols. Life Extension has a first-rate option.

Safety and Side Effects: if you stay within the recommended dosage of up 400 IU per day, from all sources, including food and supplementation, vitamin E is not known to cause any side effects. However, it is possible that vitamin E oil may cause skin irritation. Discontinue *'topical'* application and see your health care provider if soreness persists for more than 72 hours.

(4) Zinc

Zinc: is one of the most important minerals for the thymus gland and proper immune function. When zinc levels are low, so are T-cells, thymus hormone, and white blood cells. As zinc levels decline with age, its effects can largely be reversed with zinc supplements. Even the slightest zinc deficiency affects the immune system. A severe deficiency renders it chronically depressed. Anecdotal evidence from numerous health blogs supports the importance of *oral* and *topical* zinc treatment for cold sores and Genital Herpes. Topically, zinc salts inactivate the herpes viruses on contact. http://bit.ly/2rP5ogB

Zinc can be considered as part of an overall immune-enhancing program for those with recurrent herpes simplex infections. However, long-term zinc supplementation should be carefully monitored by your health-care provider and accompanied by a copper supplement. Zinc is a primary copper antagonist, which means when zinc is deficient, copper tends to accumulate in various storage organs. While too much zinc will deplete copper, both conditions can wreak havoc within the body with unexplained chronic symptoms. Fatigue is common.

Safety and Side Effects: Too much Zinc can impair instead of benefit immune function. To be safe, keep intake between 40 to 60 mg a day during outbreaks, and only 15 to 25 mg during recovery. To avoid stomach upset, take Zinc supplements with food. Besides inhibiting copper absorption, Zinc also competes with iron, calcium, and magnesium. A multi-vitamin-mineral helps prevent imbalances from taking zinc for extended periods. Another reason it's important to do a HTMA, Hair Tissue Mineral Analysis.

Zinc Arginate with Aspartate: by Advance Research is a combination designed to penetrate the cell and deliver the zinc into the plasma and inner layer of the outer cell membrane. Formulated by Hans Nieper, MD, http://bit.ly/2E0hbgM from Hannover, Germany, a physicist, and German physician, he worked as a consultant to Memorial Sloan Kettering in the 1970s.

Zinc Sulfate: is a topical form with no known side effects when used as prescribed. An application of a 0.01 to 0.025% zinc sulfate solution is effective in both reducing symptoms and inhibiting recurrences of HSV infection. Zinc lozenges can also be used to protect or inhibit the effects of the common cold or flu.

Zinc nasal sprays should be avoided: There have been reports of long lasting or permanent loss of smell.

Possible Indicator of zinc deficiency: white spots on fingernails. People with gastrointestinal disorders, malignancies, chronic illnesses, alcoholism, vegetarians, and pregnant or lactating women are all risks for poor zinc absorption. The following symptoms can indicate a need for testing, supplementing, or the very least a discussion with your health care provider:

1. Delayed wound healing.
2. Taste & smell disorders.
3. Impaired growth & sexual development.
4. Hyperactivity.
5. Impaired Adrenal Function (including stress, anxiety).

6. Skin disorders.
7. Irritable Bowel Syndrome.
8. Vision Degeneration.
9. Iron non-responsive anemia.
10. Eating disorders (such as anorexia, bulimia).

The problem with traditional lab methods is that they are not indicative of zinc's physiological cell levels. Besides the Hair Tissue Mineral Analysis (HTMA), there is a simple DIY taste test. First reported in *The Lancet*, this test uses Premier Research Labs Liquid Zinc Assay. It's an easily absorbed form of zinc sulfate to determine the body's needs. If zinc is deficient, the liquid will taste like water with adequate levels, bitter. See guide below. **The Liquid Zinc Assay** product is often "out of stock" because of demand.

Zinc Levels Taste Response:

1. **OPTIMAL:** an immediate, unpleasant taste.
2. **ADEQUATE:** immediate strong unpleasant taste that increases with time.
3. **DEFICIENT:** initially no taste but develops in 10-15 seconds.
4. **VERY DEFICIENT:** tasteless or "tastes like water."

This non-invasive test gives important feedback about the body's current zinc nutritional status. It is a form of biofeedback that can provide more accurate information than complex laboratory analysis. http://bit.ly/2DPk7tz

(5) Selenium

Frequent herpes outbreaks, the trace mineral selenium should be taken every day. Perhaps, less well known are the implications of a selenium deficiency. Research has confirmed that a *"deficiency causes flu viruses to mutate into more dangerous forms."* http://bit.ly/2nrZwEr

Selenium protects the body against oxidative damage, but a deficiency can allow benign viruses to mutate and damage the heart. Considered an antiviral, it is a great immune booster. It works in concert with iodine, and neither is efficient without the other. *"Supplementing with selenium drastically reduced the incidence of hepatitis B in both animals and humans. A clue to selenium's crucial role in immune system support is the fact that serum levels of this mineral are the single most important nutrient factor accounting for survival in AIDS patients."* http://bit.ly/2DNbvro *Biological Trace Element Research* found that **two-hundred mcg a day of selenium** increased the activity of natural killer cells by eighty-two-percent! http://bit.ly/2nmh2en The best food source for selenium is the Brazil nut. **IMPORTANT:** too much selenium can cause neurological problems. Staying under the upper tolerable limit of 400-mcg per day is important. .

B. Immune Balancing

The immune system's primary role is to protect the body against infections. Supporting and enhancing the immune system is perhaps the most crucial step we can take to keep Genital Herpes dormant. This involves a health-promoting lifestyle, stress management, exercise, diet, and the appropriate use of the following immune supporting complements.

Thymic Protein A

Nutrient deficiency is the most frequent cause of a depressed immune system. Part of that deficit is exasperated by eating copious amounts of sugar, one of the most damaging and toxic foods for the immune system. Taking a good multi-vitamin/mineral, in addition to specific supplements, can offset nutrient deficiency. http://bit.ly/2npiCv2

The thymus gland is located directly behind the sternum and is crucial for proper immune function. Like many things in life, it shrinks as we age. By our seventies, it's little more than a fatty afterthought. Fortunately, the gland produces most of the T cells (Thymus Cells) by the time we graduate from high school. The T4 (CD4) Helper Cell is the primary manager of our immune system, but it needs thymic protein to be activated.

To help stimulate T-Lymphocytes, immune compromised individuals often take **Thymic Protein A** to restore T-Lymphocytes, and the immune system's ability to fight Genital Herpes infections. *"In a randomized, placebo-controlled study, immunodeficient patients with recurrent HSV1 cold sores who were given bovine thymus extract (Thymostimulin) for six months had only 17 recurrences versus 62 in the control group. A significant increase in total white blood cells, lymphocyte count, and T-cell numbers was detected. Thymus extract may be useful in reducing the risk of viral reactivation in people who have weakened immune systems (Aiuti F et al 1984)."*

Terry Beardsley, PhD, an immunologist, and experimental biologist, discovered a biologically *"intact"* 500-amino chain protein that fits into T-4 cells receptor sites to fight disease. **He** called his discovery **Thymic Protein A (TPA).** With its unique oral delivery system, degradation is avoided in the stomach. In 1997 Dr. Beardsley was awarded a U.S. patent for both the *Thymic Protein A* molecule, and its method of production. Four micrograms of *Thymic Protein A* can be effective in strengthening our immune system against herpes infections. Benefits of Thymic Protein A include increased stamina, energy, and well-being. It's available over-the-counter.

Nutrition Review: Dr. Julian Whitaker http://bit.ly/2nqXQvb Thymic Protein A *"is likely the most powerful natural stimulant of the immune system ever discovered."* When ailing with herpes lesions, he recommends taking three packets a day sublingually. For a maintenance dose, one packet a day will help support an impaired immune system. Thymic Protein A is safe, with no adverse side effects noted in any dose.

Beta 1, 3 Glucan

The Problem: with orthodox antiviral medications, like **Acyclovir** or **Valtrex**, they target the herpes virus only when it starts replicating. Long-term regimen is often necessary to keep Genital Herpes under control. Antiviral meds kill the infected cells but killing a neuron to get rid of herpes is like *"burning down a village to save it."* A better approach would be to destroy the virus in its latent state, before it starts replicating and without damaging the infected cell. That's where beta glucan can help. Technically, beta glucan is what is called an *"immunomodulator."* It renders the immune system more successful in fighting herpes. Beta glucan does NOT *stimulate* the immune system the way Thymic Protein A stimulates T-Lymphocytes but *modulates* or *activates* the system.

Dr. Vaclav Vetvicka, PhD: in his book on beta glucan said, *"There are other agents that stimulate the immune system. However, glucans are in a class apart, because those other agents can push the immune system to overstimulation. This means they can make matters worse in the case of auto-immune illnesses such as lupus, multiple sclerosis, rheumatoid arthritis, allergies, and yeast functions."*

Beta glucan is a safe all-natural fiber molecule and the most studied natural immunomodulator on the planet. It has many benefits, not only helping the immune system do a better job keeping herpes dormant, but also stopping other diseases from establishing a foothold in the body. In an interview, Dr. Vetvicka www.glucan.us was asked: *"So if I had cancer, or if I wanted to avoid it, which beta glucan should I buy?"* He answered: *"We found that Glucan #300 from www.TransferPoint.com in the USA was the most effective against cancer."* However, that doesn't mean other brands to treat herpes infections aren't effective. Here are some other options. http://amzn.to/2DO6tLh

Beta Glucan Studies: by universities, medical schools, teaching hospitals, and even Canada's defense department, show it to be: protective against infections, lower cholesterol, and blood sugar, reduce stress, increase antibody production, heal wounds, help radiation burns, treat diabetes, and prevent the spread of cancer.

Recent breakthroughs in manufacturing have made Beta Glucan supplements affordable to most anyone. **The only caution** is if you are a transplant patient, or immunosuppressant, do not take Beta Glucan. Otherwise, to maximize its benefits, take it on an empty stomach with water. Wait at least thirty minutes before eating or drinking. During an active Genital Herpes outbreak, take between 1,000 and 3,000 mg per day. Then back off to 300 to 1,000 mg, depending on age and immune status.

Colostrum and Lactoferrin

Lactoferrin: is a key component of bovine colostrum and is six percent of the protein in Colostrum-LD, a well-recognized and researched brand name.

Colostrum: is the *pre-milk fluid* produced by female mammals just before they give birth. Technically it's not milk, but it's often called the "first-milk" because it's obtained from the first milking after birth

Colostrum-LD: is safe, non-allergenic, and has no known side effects. It can be consumed in any quantity and is safe for adults, children, and pets. In India, where cows are still considered sacred, colostrum is delivered like regular milk. It's often the first medication people take when sick. Many immune factors found in colostrum, including lactoferrin, are also transferrable from one species to another. Which means humans can benefit from immune-rich bovine or camel colostrum. While human colostrum contains only two percent IgG, bovine contains *86% IgG*. There is a wide variety of bovine colostrum products available on Amazon in the form of powder, capsules, tablets, chewable, lozenges, liquids, creams, and sprays.

Studies in animals and humans validate consuming oral lactoferrin has beneficial effects for viral infections, including the common cold, influenza, viral gastroenteritis, and herpes. Lactoferrin reduces herpes ability to penetrate human cells. http://bit.ly/2nnQidm The FDA considers lactoferrin a food and not a supplement.

2004: a lactoferricin HSV study showed, *"that bovine lactoferricin blocks herpes simplex virus binding by competing for receptor sites on target cells. However, this is apparently not the only mechanism that accounts for its anti-HSV activity."* http://bit.ly/2DYBUSi A study in *Cellular and Molecular Life Sciences* (2005), showed that lactoferrin and a peptide derived from lactoferrin, blocked entry of HSV into cells.

Safety and Side Effects: Bovine colostrum is GRAS or *"Generally Recognized as Safe."* Humans have consumed bovine lactoferrin for thousands of years through cow's milk. Children or individuals who are hypersensitive or allergic to cow's milk, have another option in Camel Whey Protein.

Dosage: for chronic Genital Herpes it depends on the state of a person's immune system. For Colostrum LD capsules, *"it's suggested to take one to four capsules twice daily with eight ounces of water between meals."* The initial dose can be increased to achieve desired results. For children and pets: one capsule one or two times daily. Open capsules and sprinkle them into food or drink if swallowing capsules is an issue.

C. Antiviral Supplements

1. Proteolytic Enzymes
2. Lysine
3. BHT
4. Coconut Oil
5. Lugol's Iodine
6. St John's Worth
7. Garlic
8. Oregano Oil
9. Apple Cider
10. Lecithin

1. Proteolytic Enzymes

Take Proteolytic Enzymes on an empty stomach, first thing in the morning, and/or at night. They remove the "gunk" from our digestive and circulatory system. They're also therapeutic for herpes, digesting its protective protein layer that surrounds the virus. Eliminating their "armor" leaves the virus unprotected and vulnerable to destruction by the immune system.

Remember: do not take proteolytic enzymes if nursing or pregnant, have a history of ulcers, or take blood thinners. If there is any intestinal discomfort, or discomfort of any kind, back down or stop altogether until the symptoms subside. If in doubt, contact your health care provider.

2. Lysine

The amino acid L-lysine is recognized as a universal treatment for herpes infections by creating antibodies and disease-fighting cells. While research is inconsistent, many bloggers rate Lysine as effective. However, better results seem to be achieved treating cold sores, rather than Genital Herpes. Used regularly, it appears to reduce the frequency and intensity of cold sores. It may be worth using Lysine for Genital Herpes to see if it helps reduce recurrent outbreaks.

If cold sores aren't upsetting enough, there's now a growing body of evidence implicating it in the development of Alzheimer's dementia (AD). http://bit.ly/2E31DsW Lysine is also under consideration as part of the AD protocol to stop the replication of HSV-1 in the brain. http://bit.ly/2nnyRK3

Suggested Lysine dose during a Genital Herpes outbreak is:

1. **Between 1500 and 2000 mg per day**, and then
2. **500 mg for daily maintenance.**

Try taking Lysine on an empty stomach rather than with food because side effects may include diarrhea, nausea, and abdominal pain. The herpes virus requires the amino acid L-Arginine to replicate properly. Lysine has a similar structure to Arginine but antagonizes its effects, making it difficult for the virus to replicate. Diets rich in Lysine and low in Arginine have been shown to help suppress HSV replication. Lysine rich foods include yogurt, fish, potatoes, and brewer's yeast. Knowing that L-Arginine promotes outbreaks, cut back on herpes' "favorite" snack foods: chocolate, peas, nuts, and seeds.

Lysine is necessary for:

1. Proper immune function,
2. Creating antibodies to fight illnesses,
3. Resistance against diseases and infections,
4. Healing skin tissue and wound healing,
5. Building collagen in the skin,
6. Functions of the heart muscle,
7. Lowers 'bad' cholesterol levels, and
8. Assists bone repair in osteoporosis.

Gelatin is rich in **Arginine**, the same amino acid that in some people aggravates herpes. Many Vitamin Capsules are made from gelatin, informally called gel-caps, manufactured from collagen of animal skin or bones. It's not required by law to list gelatin on labels, so you may need to call the manufacturer.

Lysine was the subject of the largest ever U.S. price-fixing court case, with a whopping One-Hundred-Million-dollar settlement. A few scoundrels even served prison time. They made a movie of it in 2009. You might remember, *The Informant,* starring Matt Damon. He played an L-Lysine undercover amino-acid trying to bring the Arginine-thugs to justice. *"Well, not quite the plot, but almost."* YouTube movie here http://bit.ly/2Eqp5hu.

Speaking of celebrities, Sheldon Cooper shows the love for L-Lysine when he named it his *"favorite amino acid"* on Season Two, Episode 13 of the nerdy science sitcom, *"The Big Bang Theory."* Watch the 16-second YouTube clip http://bit.ly/2DQ3GRQ.

Potential Lysine Side Effects: mainly gastric and stomach issues with diarrhea, although foods rich in Lysine do not seem to have the same effect. Kidney disease has also been linked to Lysine supplements. Again, patients with kidney and liver impairment should be cautious with any supplement, including Lysine. While L-Lysine benefits herpes infections, there is some evidence it can increase the viral load of HIV patients. For this reason, those infected with HIV/AIDS should check with their doctor first. Lysine *cannot* be produced by the body and must be consumed in food or supplement form.

3. BHT (Butylated Hydroxytoluene)

BHT is FDA Approved: as a food preservative and has a long history of benefits against the herpes virus, covered in detail by Mann and Fowke's in **'Wipe Out Herpes with BHT.'** Click the link http://bit.ly/2DLXudo to download your free copy. In animal and laboratory tests, BHT proved itself an effective agent against all lipid-coated viruses, but there are few human studies. I wonder why?

Many have claimed success using BHT to keep their cold sores and genital lesions dormant. Others have had mixed results. Because BHT is a fat-soluble additive, some recommend taking it with coconut oil, while others are just as adamant about taking it on an empty stomach. Heavier people need a higher dose. Those with little body fat need less. A typical dose of BHT ranges from one-hundred to three-hundred milligrams (100 mg to 350 mg) once or twice a day with some water on an empty stomach. If it causes stomach upset, try taking it with some coconut oil. A regular multi-vitamin can be taken with BHT, as can L-lysine and also five-hundred to one-thousand milligrams (500-1000 mg) of vitamin C. Other than that, it's recommended BHT be used as a standalone treatment. High dose vitamin C is not recommended, and grapefruit juice, colloidal silver, hydrogen peroxide and MSM are also contraindicated.

Side Effects: a common side effect of BHT is dizziness, but *"it may also cause nausea, vomiting, and stomach pain."* Start with one-hundred mg and increase the dose slowly. **IMPORTANT:** do NOT DRINK ALCOHOL while taking BHT.

BHT is potent. Careful dosing is required. For those who weigh one-hundred-twenty-five pounds (125 lbs.) or less, use no more than two-hundred-and-fifty milligrams (250 mg) of BHT per day. If you weigh two-hundred pounds (200 lbs.) the recommended dosage is five-hundred milligrams (500 mg) per day. These are guidelines. A person's age, weight, and fat content also needs to be considered. If an adverse reaction occurs, lower the dosage. More is not better. Finding the right dose can be trial and error. Especially for those aged fifty and older who are thin. *"If you choose to try this treatment always lower the amount of BHT if adverse reactions occur."*

I used BHT from January until May 2017, with the **"*Banerji*"** Protocol. BHT reduced but did not eliminate Genital Herpes outbreaks. Although BHT lacks formal scientific studies, there is a universe of anecdotal and unverified herpes success stories on blogs and forums www.EarthClinic.com. Again, the most complete BHT resource for herpes is Mann and Fowke's *"Wipe Out Herpes with BHT."* BHT is an over-the-counter supplement, but please consult with your health care provider if you have health issues or a compromised liver or kidneys. There is a large internet presence of hepatitis patients who use BHT to help improve their disease. Oscar's BHT Hepatitis blog www.EarthClinic.com can be found at, http://bit.ly/2nr17KQ.

4. Coconut Oil

Prior to the 1900s Coconut Oil was the main dietary fat in the United States. Heart disease was uncommon, and still is in countries where it's widely used.

Fast Forward to August 2018, and the American Heart Association (AHA) is still bashing coconut oil via its saturated fat content to reduce cardiovascular disease. Their claims simply don't stand up to the **research**. The AHA continues to reference faulty studies from the 1960s and 1970s that saturated fat causes heart disease (it doesn't) and that all saturated fats are the same (they're not). More importantly, studies have shown that coconut oil is anti-inflammatory, anti-microbial, and *anti-Genital Herpes*. I addition, coconut oil may actually protect against Alzheimer's disease as opposed to being a causative agent. To sum up all the coconut bashing propaganda: don't stress about eating coconut oil. The stress is more likely to give you an out-break.

Dr. Bruce Fife: a certified nutritionist, naturopathic physician, and author of more than twenty books, including *The Coconut Oil Miracle* and *Coconut Cures*, is also the director of the www.CoconutResearchCenter.org and represents the southern Colorado chapter of the Weston A. Price Foundation. According to Fife, you can *"use coconut oil to lose weight, beautify the skin and hair, prevent heart disease, cancer, diabetes, strengthen the immune system, and kill viruses that cause AIDS, influenza, hepatitis, herpes, and more."* And even though coconut oil and monolaurin have strong antiviral properties, the question remains, *"Will coconut oil prevent Genital Herpes outbreaks?"* The long and short answer, *"Yes, and maybe."*

The battle cry of most critics remains, *"Show me the evidence."* Start with www.pubmed.gov and depending on which search term you enter, there are anywhere between ten to seventeen thousand (10,000 to 17,000) research articles related to the benefits of coconut oil. To read a truncated version click http://bit.ly/2E0Vuxj.

TV personality Dr. Oz did his research. As a result, he dedicated several segments of his show to coconut oil's many benefits. In 2022 he's running for a seat in the U.S. Senate from Pennsylvania. http://bit.ly/2FttI9C. To fight Genital Herpes, he recommends combining oral consumption with topical application. It can also be used as cooking oil, butter, and added to that morning cup of "super" java. Delicious! The only caution is to build-up internal consumption slowly. Coconut oil has many immune-stimulating and antioxidant properties. It supports thermogenesis (heat) and increases metabolism by nourishing the thyroid and our cells mitochondrial function. Two thirds of coconut oil consist of Medium Chain Triglycerides (MCTs). These MCTs contain three healthy fatty acids with proven anti-microbial and herpes properties:

1. **Lauric Acid** (40 – 50%)
2. **Capric Acid** (7 – 10%)
3. **Caprylic Acid** (about 8%)

They are powerful antimicrobial agents, effective against a wide range of bacteria, viruses, fungi, yeasts, and protozoa. Two factors seem critical for herpes treatment:

1. **The quantity** needed to achieve therapeutic levels of lauric acid, and
2. **How much** lauric acid converts into monolaurin to be effective.

Weston A. Price Foundation: www.WestonAPrice.org, suggests eating as much coconut oil as possible to maximize lauric acid levels in the body. Other health advocates recommend starting with two-to-three (2-to-3) tablespoons and increasing the dosage until symptoms subside. Results appear mixed. Many claim positive results, just as many discouraging outcomes. **Dr. Jon Kabara,** credited with discovering the antimicrobial effects of monoglycerides, believes the body converts only a small amount of coconut oil into monolaurin. Not enough for a therapeutic response against herpes.

Kabara Claims: the body needs three-to-nine (3-to-9) grams of monolaurin a day for an antiviral effect. That's eating three-thousand to nine-thousand milligrams (3000 to 9000 mg) of coconut oil a day. Not sure if most people want to or even can force down 2-to-3 cups of coconut oil. It might start leaking out their bottom. To get an effective amount of monolaurin, perhaps it's best to take it in supplement form. A single dose of *Lauricidin* is the equivalent of many tablespoons of coconut oil.

What is Lauricidin? It's the brand name supplement of pure sn-1 monolaurin derived from coconut oil. It was designed to replace copious amounts of coconut oil needed to kill the herpes virus on contact. Lauricidin can also be used as a cream for topical application. It is safe and many swear by it. There are thousands of testimonials that claim Lauricidin stopped or greatly reduced their Genital Herpes outbreaks. However, it may need to be taken every day to maintain its effectiveness. There have been no reported negative side effects from long-term use. LAURICIDIN® is more cost-effective when purchased directly from the manufacturer at www.Lauricidin.com.

If initial levels are too high, a person can experience short-term, flu-like symptoms:

1. Headaches,
2. Body aches,
3. Acne, itchy skin, and mild rashes,
4. Skin flushing,
5. Sore throat,
6. General malaise, and
7. Sweating, chills, and/or nausea.

Temporary Herxheimer reactions are common, and normal, even healthy. Studies showed Monolaurin supplements reduced Genital Herpes outbreaks, but individual outcomes vary.

5. Lugol's Iodine

Iodine: is required by every tissue in our body, but especially our thyroid. It's often called *the endocrine mineral* because of its importance to the thyroid, adrenals, ovaries, breasts, and prostate. **Lugol's Iodine** can be used internally or topically on herpes sores. Internal consumption depends on each person's tolerance and deficiency. For Genital Herpes, start with a topical five-to-ten (5-to-10) drops of two-and-a-half percent (2.5%) Lugol's solution on the inner thighs, sacrum, and/or stomach area. Also, apply a small dab directly to herpes lesions once or twice a day. If it stings, dilute it with distilled water. Also, unless you are a dolphin or fisherman who only eats seaweed and fish, you're deficient. And, if you decide to eat only fish and seaweed, you will probably die at an early age from mercury poisoning.

So, what to do? First, do your research. But please don't just listen to the *"so called"* experts that claim people get enough iodine from food. They're wrong. Iodine deficiency is associated with cancers, strokes, and other serious health problems.

There is an *iodine deficiency epidemic*. It effects almost every man, woman, and child, but especially vegetarians. Over the past thirty to forty (30 to 40) years, iodine intake in the U.S. has declined by more than fifty percent (50%), while increasing amounts of competing, toxic halogens of bromine, fluorine, and chlorine have found their way into our food supply. For example, iodine in wheat has been replaced with bromine, the same gas used to fumigate termites in your home. Most iodine resides in the sea or seashore. Unless you live in Laguna Beach or Catalina Island, eat fish every day, odds are you're deficient. Contributing factors:

1. Diets low in fish,
2. Vegan diets,
3. Poor iodine availability in commercial salt,
4. Toxic farming techniques,

5. Avoiding sea-salt for fear of high blood pressure,
6. Ingesting toxic halogens, and the increased use of
7. Radioactive iodine in medical procedures (competes with natural iodine).

In addition, past food sources of iodine have been removed. From the 1960s to the 1980s, iodide was used as a dough conditioner in baked goods, but it's been replaced with bromide, a toxic halogen.

Symptoms? Brittle nails, cold hands and feet, depression, difficulty swallowing, dry skin, dry hair or hair loss, fatigue, high cholesterol, hoarseness, infertility, lethargy, menstrual irregularities, early menopause, poor memory or concentration, slower heartbeat, throat pain, weight gain, and yes, frequent herpes outbreaks. If so, iodine deficiency, and/or being hypothyroid might warrant a consideration.

Two forms: iodine and iodide. The thyroid mainly uses iodide. Dr. Lugol's solution is five-percent (5%) iodine and ten-percent (10%) potassium iodide in water to increase solubility. Two drops of Lugol's five percent (5%) solution in water contains about twelve-and-half milligrams (12.50 mg) of iodine/iodide daily. The Japanese daily iodine intake averages about *thirteen-point-eight milligrams* (13.8 mg), or about one-hundred (100) times the U.S. RDA. They have lower rates of breast, endometrial and ovarian cancer, and significantly lower rates of fibrocystic breast disease and prostate cancer. The prevalence of herpes in Japan is also far lower compared to that of the United States. Sometimes association is the cause.

6. St John's Wort

St. John's Worth is a strong antiviral substance, so it should be implemented with some degree of caution and with the advice a health care provider knowledgeable with natural medicine. There are two options: taking St. John's Wort as a dietary supplement, and/or applying the oil directly to herpes blisters. Both types of St. John's Wort supplements can be found online or at an organic health food store. You can try the recommended dosage for three (3) months as part of your Genital Herpes elimination strategy.

7. Garlic

Dracula, Bram Stokers used garlic to repel vampires. The ancient Egyptians worshipped garlic as a "minor" god, and on occasion used it as local currency. Hippocrates, the father of medicine, was more practical. He used it to treat and heal infections. Since ancient time garlic has been known to kill bacteria, fungus, and viruses. Today, it may deter Genital Herpes and candida. Numerous studies reported favorable results and therapeutic effects of treating herpes with garlic. Scientists have succeeded in killing the herpes virus in laboratory conditions. The key phrase, *"laboratory conditions."* http://bit.ly/2DO4gvo

Like herpes: garlic is also no slouch. It contains thirty-three (33) sulfur compounds, every essential amino acid, all major minerals, several trace minerals, as well as vitamins A, B, and C. But the chemicals allicin and ajoene are what makes garlic effective against HSV-1 or HSV-2. In 1992, Planta Medica published a study that used fresh garlic juice on several different viruses. Garlic destroyed ninety percent (90%) of any virus within thirty (30) minutes. In their scientific paper, they recommended that people use the following garlic protocol for its antiviral herpetic benefits. http://bit.ly/2nq9U0j

1. Eat **one** teaspoon of fresh minced "raw" garlic every day for prevention.
2. Eat **two** teaspoons at the first sign of an infection.

Allicin is that spicy, scorching, smelly stuff that makes garlic such a powerhouse in a crowded bus or bloodstream. I'm not a huge fan of garlic supplements because of their expense, and they don't appear to work as well. A garlic press, some peeled garlic, and a bit of Witherspoon's raw honey may be a better carrier option.

SIDE EFFECTS: according to www.WebMd.com, *"Garlic has been used safely for up to seven years. When taken by mouth, garlic can cause bad breath, a burning sensation in the mouth or stomach, heartburn, gas, nausea, vomiting, body odor, and diarrhea. Garlic may also increase the risk of bleeding."*

8. Oregano Oil

Oregano essential oil for Genital Herpes:

1. Helps prevent outbreaks.
2. Reduces severity of symptoms.
3. Settles down lesions.
4. Protects against fungus and bacteria.
5. Not cheap, but affordable, and
6. Suitable for both internal and topical use.

Oregano Oil: can relieve the pain and itching of Genital Herpes, accelerate the healing process, and prevent spreading infections. Extracted from the oregano herb, it is an effective free-radical-destroying antioxidant, and a potent antibiotic. Oregano's primary active compound is **carvacrol.** The higher the percentage (85%) of carvacrol, the greater its antiviral properties. It also contains *origanum heracleoticum,* which keeps bacterial strains under control. Oregano oil breaks down the lipid bilayer of the herpes cell membrane, then penetrates the virus and destroys it. Oregano is successful because it inhibits the virus at various stages of infection and replication, and helps the immune system inhibit viral transmission to another host.

Multiple studies, including from the **U.S. Department of Agriculture**, reported, *"oregano oil has such a strong action against germs that it easily fights Salmonella and E. coli."* One study examined the relationship between oregano oil and harmful organisms and found that taking 600 mg of oregano oil daily prompted a complete disappearance of harmful organisms in the body. Oregano oil is available in capsule or liquid form. Make sure to purchase high-quality oil. Here are some things to consider when evaluating oregano oil:

1. Most oregano oils contain somewhere between fifty to eighty-five (50 to 85) percent of carvacrol. The more potent, the more expensive.

2. Avoid additional fillers and solvents. Instead, look for unprocessed, raw, steam distilled, and undiluted oils.

Topical Application: it's 'essential' to dilute oregano oil. Some products come pre-diluted (25% oregano oil), but for *sensitive* individuals or children it may need to be diluted further. To dilute one-hundred percent (100%) oregano, add a *"carrier oil."* Coconut oil, olive oil, or castor oil are quality oils. To make a twenty-five percent (25%) concentration of oregano oil, add one-part oregano to three-parts carrier oil. Test a small skin area before using it on Genital Herpes sores.

Never Use: oregano oil or any essential oil in the eyes or ears. If oregano oil inflames the skin, apply more coconut or castor oil, and dilute more. If it accidentally gets into your eyes, add *"full-fat-milk"* or castor oil to the eye.

Internal consumption: dilute oregano oil before swallowing or absorbing it under the tongue. Methods to consume oregano oil drops:

1. Hold oregano drops under the tongue.
2. Put drops into an empty Vitamin Capsule, or
3. Mix oil drops into two-ounce (2-oz). full-fat milk.

Start with a two-drop dose. It's strong! If you have a twenty-five percent (25%) oregano oil solution, eight (8) drops of diluted oregano oil will equal two drops of pure oil. The oil can irritate the stomach. Taking it with a bit of coconut oil or fatty food is ideal. There are also commercial gel-cap preparations available on Amazon. Adding drops of oregano oil to a glass of water is NOT a promising idea. The oil will float on top and burn the lips or mouth. It does not dilute or dissolve in water!

There are overpriced products sold through personal distributors. While they are of high quality, less expensive but similar oils are available online. Oregano oil offers a lot when it comes to fighting herpes. Used both internally and externally, it's a safe and effective option to say goodbye and wave bon-voyage to the herpes titanic.

9. Apple Cider Vinegar (ACV)

Benefits: raw, unfiltered ACV is a fermented food, *"like sauerkraut, kefir, kimchi and kombucha. Its cloudy appearance and cobweb strings means the vinegar is living and full of nutrients. The strings are the mother, like kefir grains used to ferment kefir. If there is no mother, there would be no vinegar."* www.EarthClinic.com Raw ACV is made from apples, nothing else. They are crushed into fresh apple cider and allowed to ferment.

Apple Cider Vinegar: the Ph is at times confusing. It helps alkalize the body, yet it has a pH of three, which is acidic. However, raw ACV improves mineral balance and digestion, which alkalizes the body. An acidic body is at a higher risk for sickness and a prolonged healing process, including Genital Herpes. Acidity has been linked to many health problems, including cancer. Watch Earth Clinic's founder Deirdre Layne make an ACV and baking soda tonic here http://bit.ly/2GzeYHC.

On the other side of the isle, grocery store vinegars are heated, filtered, and pasteurized. They look sterile and transparent compared to Bragg's Organic unfiltered ACV with the *mother*. Depending on how it's used, grocery store vinegar is OK for some external applications, such as a fungal foot soak. But for internal consumption, please use only organic, raw ACV.

Raw ACV for Genital Herpes: decreases the severity of outbreaks because of its disinfectant, astringent, and anti-inflammatory properties. It can be used topically or internally.

Topical ACV

For Genital Herpes, dilute raw ACV with an equal amount of distilled water. Dip a cotton ball into the ACV and dab it on the affected areas three or four times a day. For the best results, apply at the first sign or initial tingling sensation. Be aware, it's going to sting, but it'll calm down. The acid in the vinegar quickly goes to work removing excess oil and drying out the sores and lesions. If a 50/50 solution feels comfortable, try a stronger blend the next day until the lesions heal. Repeat this remedy until signs of improvement.

Internal ACV

Ingesting ACV is for prevention. Several options and protocols to consider.

Breakfast: add two teaspoons of raw unfiltered ACV to a clean glass of water. Consume first thing in the morning before breakfast. This regular health tonic can help strengthen the gut flora and body's immune system, while keeping herpes dormant.

Lunch & Dinner: add two tablespoons of ACV into a sixteen-ounce (16 oz.) empty glass bottle, then mix in a quarter (¼) teaspoon of baking soda. Wait until the fizzing stops and fill with clean, pure water. Drink half during lunch, and the other half with dinner. It's best to start low-and-slow with one or two teaspoons and then increase the amount over time. For certain acute conditions, or chronic Genital Herpes outbreaks, more can be taken at any time. The range of health conditions that ACV benefits is truly staggering. Here is a brief list of diseases that have benefited from raw ACV:

1. Heartburn
2. **Herpes**
3. Reflux
4. Shingles
5. Warts
6. Eczema
7. Bladder infections
8. Nail fungus
9. Constipation
10. High Blood Pressure
11. Sinus Infection
12. Gout
13. Diabetes
14. Gall bladder attacks
15. Leg cramps
16. Arthritis
17. Flu
18. Colds

Maybe ACV belongs in your medicine cabinet, not the kitchen cabinet. But like all treatments, ACV may not be the perfect remedy for everyone. While it works for many, for some it causes side effects. It's OK to start with a lesser amount and increase the dosage slowly until a desired effect is obtained.

10. Hydrogen Peroxide

Hydrogen Peroxide (H_2O_2) therapy has many benefits. It helps eliminate infections, reduces pain, and detoxes the body. Topical hydrogen peroxide is a popular home remedy for Genital Herpes. H_2O_2 is nothing more than oxygen and water combined in a ratio to form a germicidal liquid.

When hydrogen peroxide is taken as an internal remedy, it reacts with organic material and breaks down into water and oxygen. The added oxygen in the body creates an environment where most "microbes," including Genital Herpes, cannot flourish or survive. Oxidation serves as a fundamental objective in restoring well-being and relieving illness.

Topical application: take a cotton ball and apply a three percent (3%) H2O2 solution to the infected area. Leave it on for a few minutes, then wipe or wash off. Repeat this process every few hours for a couple of days. For an added benefit, open a Lysine capsule and mix it with hydrogen peroxide, then apply. For oral sores, or as a mouthwash, start with a mixture of one-part hydrogen peroxide and three parts distilled water. Gargle or swish a few times a day for two or three days. Increase the hydrogen peroxide percentage until it feels uncomfortable.

Internal Consumption: according to the FDA, oral H2O2 might cause gastrointestinal irritation or ulcers. Yes, so does ibuprofen. But most people aren't foolish enough to take ten (10) ibuprofens or swallow a quart of peroxide. According to EarthClinic, the standard dose for food grade peroxide is three-to-four (3-4) drops in an eight-ounce (8 oz.) glass of water. http://bit.ly/2nv4Mrf *Hydrogen Peroxide Therapy: Benefits and Side Effects*. **WARNING: never use** food grade thirty-five-percent (35%) H2O2 solution topically. Please visit EarthClinic at the link above, for a detailed outline if you wish to pursue internal consumption.

11. Lecithin

Nerves are coated with a fatty insulation called the myelin sheath. This sheath acts like the rubber lining around an electrical wire to prevent interference and keeps the energy flowing. Lecithin may be helpful in preserving the integrity of the myelin sheath and combating the deterioration of the nerve pathways caused by Genital Herpes outbreaks.

Lecithin is a non-toxic fatty compound occurring naturally in animal and plant tissues. Many blogs support the use of Lecithin supplements to stop Genital Herpes outbreaks. In addition, it is said to be useful to control eczema. Hospitals use lecithin-based formula's on newborn babies whose mothers have Genital Herpes.

Anecdotal evidence on many blogs suggests taking between two-and-four-thousand milligrams (2000 - 4000 mg) a day for thirty days to prevent outbreaks. I recommend a Non-GMO Sunflower Lecithin versus Soy Lecithin. You can purchase Lecithin in powder of gel caps. The author has no experience using this supplement in relationship to herpes

D. Topical Antivirals

1. Essential Oils

Oregano, Clove, Tea Tree, and Myrrh are four popular oils that support the Genital Herpes healing process. Start with Tea Tree. It has natural antiviral and bacterial properties and can be applied *"neat"* (undiluted) or mixed with a carrier oil. Or mix and match all four essential oils in various combinations, either *"neat"* or with a carrier oil. Experiment and see which combination works best for you. **Three options are:**

1. **Apply** each oil separately with a Q-tip, or
2. **Blend** all four "neat" in a one (1) ml jar; or
3. **Blend** in one-ounce (1 oz.) dropper bottle, add a carrier oil of choice.

For a carrier oil use either coconut, olive, or castor oil. For sensitive skin types, please patch-test oils before using them. Put a drop or two on an inner forearm to make sure there are no negative reactions. Start slow,, and if too strong, dilute them further with a carrier oil. Then apply and coat Genital Herpes sores three times daily or as needed. Remember, if you use oils 'neat' (undiluted), one-to-three (1-to-3) drops is usually sufficient. For the sacrum, you may prefer a fifty/fifty (50/50) mix with a carrier oil. For all sensitive skin areas (labia, genital, or lips) consider further dilution. Start slow, then work your way into using them neat.

2. Manuka Honey

Manuka honey delivers better results than Acyclovir ointment when treating symptoms of labial or Genital Herpes. A good brand is Wedderspoon http://bit.ly/2np8nrh raw honey for treating both cold sores and Genital Herpes. Do not use processed sugary honey found in supermarkets. In clinical studies, manuka honey effectively eradicated over two-hundred-fifty (250) strains of bacteria, including antibiotic-resistant strains. However, if the infection is serious, **Medihoney** may be a better choice. *Medihoney* is an advanced wound care dressing that promotes wound healing.

3. Lemon Balm Antiviral Cream

Lemon Balm Cream is an excellent herbal remedy for the treatment of herpes, blisters, shingles, and cold sores. The salve increases the production of skin cells to heal cold sores, shingles, and pox rashes. Regular topical use may also lessen outbreak frequency. Amazon has several options to choose from. Review their ratings, stick with those that are "natural" and have a favorable return policy.

4. Abreva Docosanol Cream

Abreva cream works for **cold sores** by penetrating the skin to the source of the virus. It claims to block the virus and provide a barrier to protect healthy skin cells. It's not intended to be used for Genital Herpes, but some HSV-2 bloggers have claimed success using it.

5. Zinc Oxide, Castor Oil Cream

Zinc helps the body produce lymphocyte cells, which can reduce herpes outbreaks and boost the immune system's ability to fight the virus. Studies show that zinc deactivates herpes and inhibits reproduction. Sores may heal up to 40% faster than leaving them to heal on their own. Zinc can relieve the pain experienced with outbreaks.

A zinc castor oil cream by "Third Day Naturals" is typically applied before bedtime, and overnight the herpes sores can shrink and dry out. If an outbreak is severe, apply the cream intermittently throughout the day, alternating with other listed options. http://bit.ly/2BHGlf5 The cream is not designed for cold sores, but as a barrier cream. However, in test tubes, zinc has been shown to be an effective agent against both HSV-1 and HSV-2. In one small study, people who applied zinc oxide cream to cold sores saw them heal faster than those who applied a placebo. **WARNING:** Zinc Oxide ointments are recommended for men but not women. Drying agents should not be used in the vaginal area. Use a Q-Tip or cotton swab to apply Zinc Oxide creams.

6. Silver Gel Cream

A potent silver gel cream from **www.SilverPure.com** can be used on herpes lesions and eczema rashes. The company creates skin creams and salves infused with **thirty-five-thousand (35,000) Parts Per Million (PPM) nano-silver particles**. There is obviously a difference between thirty-five-thousand (**35,000) Parts Per Million (PPM)** and the more common drug store twenty-five-parts-per-million (25 PPM), not only in PPMs, but effectiveness. As of this writing, their products do not contain harmful chemicals or skin irritants, only natural oils, mixed with various antioxidants. They are then infused with ten-to-thirty-five-Thousand-parts-per-thousand elemental silver nanoparticles (10,000 to 35,000 PPM), giving the creams powerful anti-microbial properties effective against bacteria, viruses, and fungi.

For thousands of years, silver was the go-to first line-of-defense against pathogens. Then patentable antibiotics hit center stage. However, unlike with antibiotics, bacteria, viruses, and fungi have not built immunity to elemental silver. In addition, silver improves healing by stimulating dermal and epidermal regeneration, while decreasing redness and inflammation. Best of all, it's non-toxic.

7. Lauricidin

Herpes is among the ten most frequently searched conditions on the internet. With so much concern, and so many looking for solutions, what are the medical *"experts"* doing? Other than to offer topical Acyclovir or antiviral drugs? Not much. Enter Lauricidin, the brand name of a high monolaurin supplement formula, designed to replace eating copious amounts of coconut oil. Please see the manufacturer's web site for more information at www.lauricidin.com. For a topical solution mix one scoop of Lauricidin into one-or-two ounces (1-or-2 oz) of medium/hot distilled water. Stir into a soft paste, and when cool, apply to blisters several times a day, or as needed.

8. MMS1 & DMSO Solution

Do a patch test inside your forearm before applying MMS1 or DMSO to your Genital Herpes lesions. Be extra cautious if you are applying it to the sensitive areas of your privates. Remember, everyone's biology is unique, and we react differently to what we put in and on our bodies. Chlorine Dioxide (MMS1) and DMSO are strong medicines. Treat them with respect. (See MMS Protocol Chapter Ten (10) for more information.)

Topical MMS Solution for Genital Herpes

1. **Add 4 drops** of un-activated MMS in a glass shooter.
2. **Add 4 drops of 4% HCL.**
3. **Wait 30 to 60 seconds** (it's now activated MMS1).
4. **Add 4 drops of 99.99% DMSO** to the solution, then
5. **Wait a minute or two,** mix in 6 drops of distilled water.
6. **Q-Tip the MMS1** mixture to your blisters.

9. Miscellaneous: two more topical Genital Herpes treatments worth of mentioning:

Lidocaine: anesthetic jelly works to reduce the pain of outbreaks and can be purchased over the counter. It also exists in (Rx) prescription strength, but you'll need a 'script' from you doctor.

Epsom Salt: is healing and soothing. Soaking your labial or genital HSV-2 lesions in Epsom salt is beneficial and keeps the area clean to prevent secondary infections. Fill a tub with about three or four (3 or 4) inches of very warm water. Add one-to-one-and-a-half cups (1 ½) or more, of Epsom salt and wait until dissolved. Sit in the solution for fifteen (15) minutes, two or three times a day. Make sure the outbreak area is fully covered. Afterwards, rinse with warm water, but do not use soap. If you have health concerns, check with your doctor. A sitz bath is a warm, shallow bath that cleanses the perineum, the area between the rectum and the vulva or scrotum. **CAUTION:** If you have low blood pressure, Adrenal Fatigue, and/or hypothyroid, please check with your health care provider before using Epsom salt (magnesium sulfate). It could lower your blood pressure further.

PART FOUR: HEALING THE MIND

"Fungus is more complicated than Herpes, they are "Eukaryotes," which means they have cells. Herpes does not."

Viruses are different from all other <u>Infectious Microorganisms</u> because they are the only group entirely reliant on a host cell (humans) for replication.

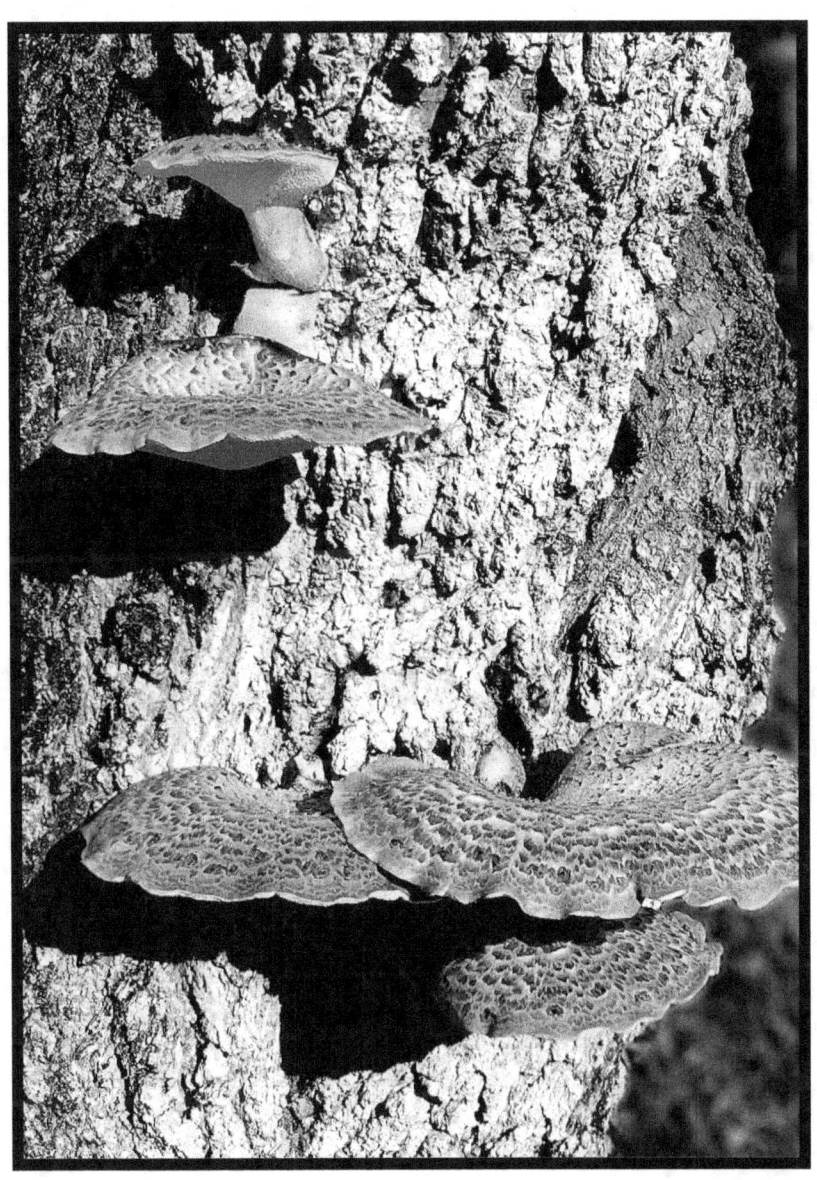

Chapter 12: Psychology of Health

Most people become interested in their health only after they've misplaced it. Then they want to quickly find it again. And who can blame them. Unfortunately, health is not like misplacing your keys or glasses. Quick solutions, instant remedies, or a pill for every illness, often end up exchanging or compounding losses even further. Please don't be like most people. If you've misplaced your health, and are out-of-sorts, we can help you find it again. But be patient, and even if it's lost forever, there are answers that'll help you find your smile again.

So, what is health? Modern medicine tells us when there is no disease, what remains is health. This is deception in the form of a truncated definition. It's like defining light in relationship to darkness, or life to death. If you're not dead, you're alive. Genius.

Medicine's dilemma? It's not qualified to tell us what health is, only disease. The irony is that most of the time they don't even know its cause. But they sure know how to treat symptoms with endless rounds of drugs, chemo, radiation, or surgery. For example, *"Most cancer patients in this country die of chemotherapy. Chemotherapy does not eliminate breast, colon, or lung cancers. This fact has been documented for over a decade, yet doctors still use chemotherapy for these tumors."* Allen Levin, MD, UCSF, *The Healing of Cancer*. **It's time** to change our approach and become more of our own health advocates.

A. EFT Tapping

Emotional Freedom Techniques: (EFT), or simply Tapping or EFT Tapping, is a form of psychological acupressure. It's based on the same energy meridians used for over 5,000 years in traditional acupuncture, but without needles. Not only does EFT work, but it also has impressive science and research http://bit.ly/2FyTtp0 to back up its claims. Take your physical and emotional well-being into your own hands with EFT. It's simple, effective, and anyone can master it. The best part, it's free.

Tapping provides relief *"from chronic pain, emotional problems, addictions, phobias, Post-Traumatic-Stress-Disorder, and most physical diseases. Like acupuncture and acupressure, the practice consists of Tapping with your fingertips on specific meridian points to release energy blockages."* http://bit.ly/2FAmGAf If herpes infections have you feeling tired, unwell, in frequent pain, depressed, or anxious, consider EFT. Tapping is one of the cornerstones of the Hermes Protocol.

*"The cause of all negative emotions is a disruption
in our body's energy system."* - Gary Craig

With EFT you *"tune in"* or focus on the issue while stimulating (Tapping) various meridian points on your body with fingertips. For most health-related issues, it reduces the conventional therapeutic process from weeks, months, or years down to minutes, hours, or days. Millions have embraced EFT worldwide. Astonishing results have been achieved for pain, diseases, emotional issues, PTSD, and performance enhancement. An original EFT Manual (now obsolete) by founder Gary Craig was translated into 23 languages and downloaded by over 2 million people worldwide. http://bit.ly/2nuOjTW

*"EFT is an emotional version of acupuncture,
except we use our fingers and not needles."* - Gary Craig

Start EFT: by first learning the locations of the energy points. They're not difficult to memorize. The diagram on the next page illustrates their points in detail. In addition, there are literally hundreds of YouTube presentations where you can simply tap along with whatever issue or subject interests you. Click here http://bit.ly/2E13Wwy for the basic recipe by EFT founder Gary Craig. EFT works both on an emotional and physical level to improve our well-being. Its intent is to find the root cause of the problem and collapse the *"beliefs and negative emotions"* that disrupt the body's energy system.

How a Negative Emotion is Caused

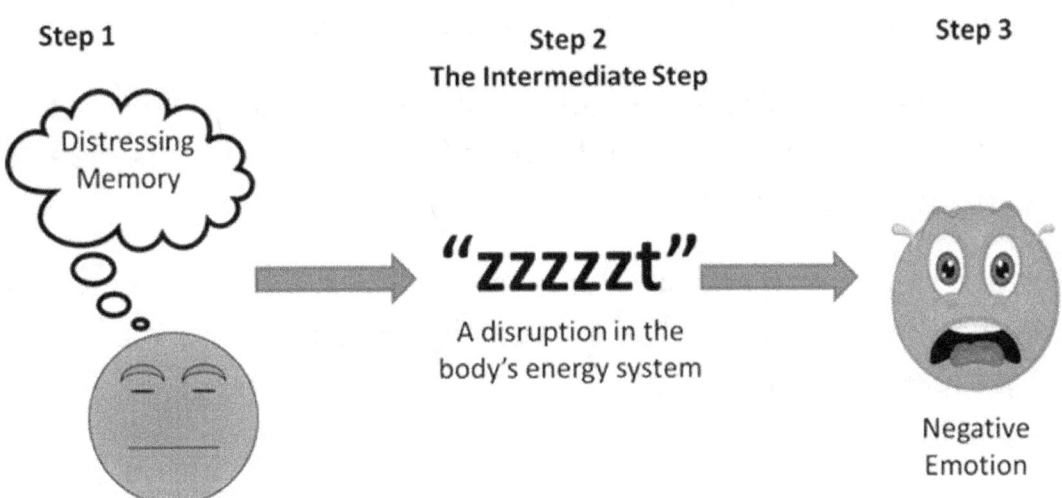

"EFT can assist physical healing by resolving
underlying energetic or emotional contributors." - Gary Craig

The theory behind EFT: is quite simple. *"Deep-rooted emotional wounds are stored in the body/mind as blocked energy patterns. Stimulating specific energy points by gently Tapping on them, while at the same time mentally focusing on them, over time releases their obstruction. As the energy is brought back into balance, thoughts about distressing circumstances change, and negative emotions diminish. This process takes place on a bio-electromagnetic level throughout our being.*

The Six-Step EFT Tapping Technique:

1. **First, Choose a problem.** For example, *"I have a Genital Herpes outbreak on my sacrum."*

2. **Rate the intensity** of your negative feeling to that problem from zero to ten (0-10) with ten (10) being the most intense. *"I rate my negative feelings, combined with the pain and discomfort as an eight (8)."*

3. **After you've rated your intensity:** state the following affirmation three times while Tapping the Karate Chop spot (see chart of Tapping Points below): *"Even though I have a Genital Herpes outbreak on my sacrum, I deeply and completely, love, honor, and accept myself."*

4. **Tap the remaining energy points:** as you speak a reminder words or a phrase such as, *"this herpes outbreak on my sacrum"*, or *"my anger/fear/guilt about my herpes outbreak on my sacrum."*

5. **Take a deep breath:** Take stock. What is your rating now? Notice any new thoughts or memories and repeat Step Four (4) as often as needed until each one is neutralized.

6. **Return to the original problem:** repeat Steps Four and Five (4 and 5) until you reach zero or the problem is resolved. Zero means you no longer feel a negative charge.

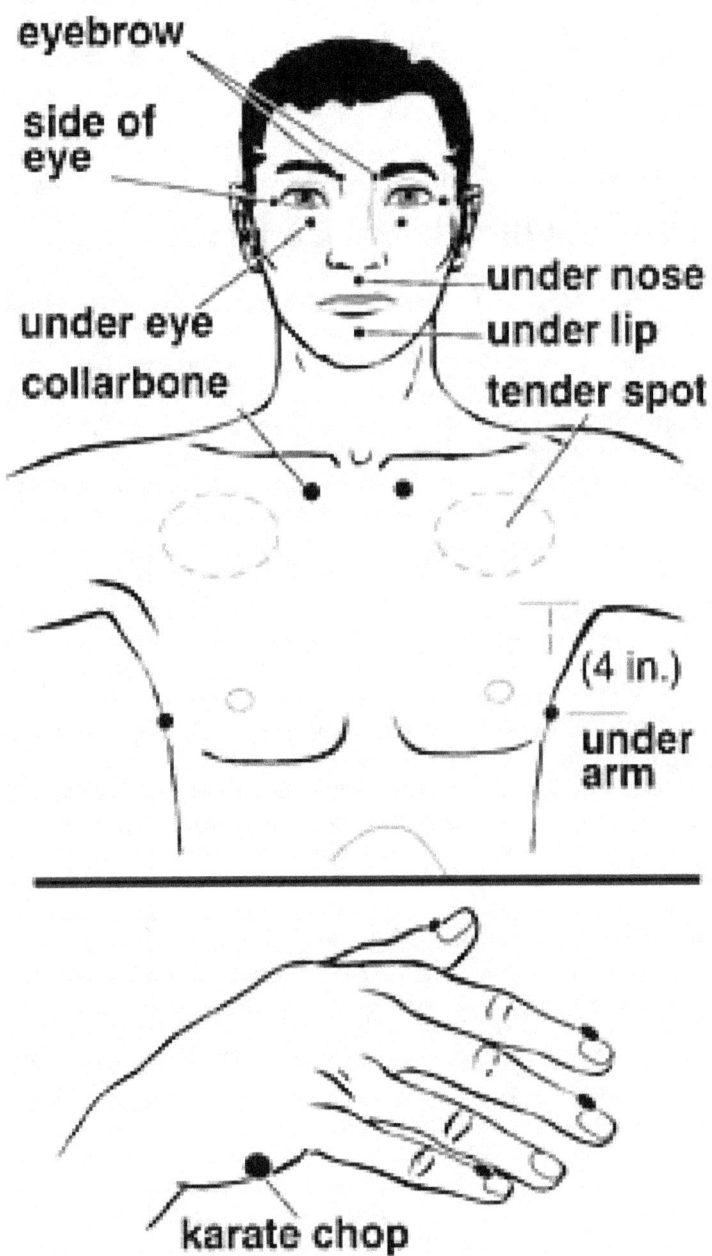

The Tapping Points and Their Meridians

1. **Karate Chop (KC):** Small Intestine Meridian, side of the hand, small finger side
2. **Beginning of Eyebrow (BE): starting point of the Bladder Meridian**
3. **Side of Eye (SE):** end-point of the Triple Warmer Meridian, beginning point of the Gall Bladder Meridian
4. **Under the Eye (UE):** Stomach Point Meridian
5. **Under Nose (UN):** end-point of the Governing Meridian
6. **Chin (CH): end-point of the Central Meridian**
7. **Collarbone (CB):** Kidney Meridian & Adrenal Gland Function
8. **Under Arm (UA):** ending point of the Spleen Meridian
9. **Top of Head (TH):** This set of points is located at the top of the head and overly sensitive. Tap gently on this area, using all your fingers.

EFT can be applied to physical symptoms without exploring an emotional cause. However, for more positive and longer lasting results, it's best to identify and target the underlying emotional issue. According to EFT, the more unresolved emotional issues a person clears, the more peace and freedom they will enjoy. Tapping, self-limiting beliefs fade, personal performance increases, relationships start to blossom, and health improves.

With that in mind, EFT is best used as an ongoing process to clear out old traumas and welcome new challenges with a healthy, positive attitude. Try EFT and see if it doesn't improve your herpes outbreaks, giving you more peace of mind and freedom.

"Over a million-people suffering through natural or human-caused disasters have been treated with EFT, according to charities that offer aid to these victims." (Capacitar, 2013; TREST, 2010; Veterans Stress Project, 2013). Something to think about when we reflect on those displaced and suffering individuals when hurricanes Irma and Harvey slammed into Texas and Florida in 2017. Be grateful, seek happiness. Not pleasure.

B. Dapper Tappers

Brad Yates is a favorite tap-along teacher with hundreds of different Tapping solutions via his website and YouTube Channel (https://bit.ly/420Xhtu) .

Three Brad Yates Tap-Along:

1. **Optimal Health:** Metabolism and Aging http://bit.ly/2E0TEg1
2. **Healing:** from the Inside Out http://bit.ly/2rWA9QS
3. **Happy Tapping:** Freeing Negativity http://bit.ly/2BHw6rf

Gary Craig, the originator of EFT, is the consummate teacher and educator. The excellence of his training is only surpassed by commitment and contributions to the EFT community. To get up to Tapping speed, visit www.emofree.com. It's Craig's Official EFT Training Center. He remains the 'go-to' resource.

1. **EFT Tapping Intro:** by Gary Craig http://bit.ly/2DPPluV
2. **EFT and Emotional Balance:** Gary Craig http://bit.ly/2E2FoTJ
3. **EFT for Serious Diseases:** Gary Craig http://bit.ly/2Fxu2Ep

Nick and Jessica Ortner, brother and sister team, have authored several bestselling books under their main title, *The Tapping Solution*. It's also their website.

1. **EFT Tapping for Pain Relief:** Nick Ortner http://bit.ly/2EtTYli
2. **Tapping Meditation:** Peace & Light Jessica Ortner http://bit.ly/2nwgOk1
3. **Nick Ortner Taps on Shoulder Pain** http://bit.ly/2BHUuJ2

C. Herpes Tapping Script

First, choose the problem. *"I have a Genital Herpes outbreak on my sacrum."*

Then tune in and rate the intensity of your negative feelings to that problem, from 0-10, with 10 being the most intense. *"I rate my negative feelings, combined with the pain and discomfort as a 7 or 8."*

After rating the intensity, state the following affirmation **at least three times** while Tapping the Karate Chop spot.

1. Side of Hand: *"Even though I have these painful herpes outbreak on my (location), I deeply and completely accept myself."*

"Even though I have all this anger in my body, I deeply and completely love, and accept myself."

"Even though I feel so sad and angry about my Genital Herpes, I deeply and completely love, honor, and accept myself." (Repeat one more time from the beginning.)

Tap the rest of the points: feeling your pain, anger, etc. in your body.

2. **Eyebrow Point:** *All this pain on my _____.*

3. **Side of Eye:** *All this pain.*

4. **Under Eye:** *It's safe to express my feelings, about herpes outbreak.*

5. **Under Nose:** *It's safe to let it all out.*

6. **Under Mouth:** *This painful Genital Herpes outbreak on my _____.*

7. **Collarbone:** *I can feel it in my body.*

8. **Under arm:** *I can express all my feelings now.*

9. **Top of Head:** *It's safe to let it all out now.*

Continue Tapping through the points again (and again), putting into words, expressing how Genital Herpes outbreak(s) affects your life, body, emotions, and state of mind. Let your feelings be on fire while Tapping through the points. See it, feel it, and if there is something to say to someone, say it aloud while Tapping through the points.

When you're ready to stop, take a deep, slow breath, and check back with how you feel. On a *"feelings"* scale of zero to ten, rate yourself again. If emotions and pain are still running high, repeat as necessary until you feel calm. Be kind to yourself, keep Tapping.

D. Medication to Meditation

"The trouble with ignorance, it picks up confidence as it goes along."

1. States of Illusion

Many, many years ago, I read a best-selling book about a woman who achieved enlightenment in Paris while getting onto a city bus. I remember thinking, *"Maybe I'm doing it all wrong. Maybe I should just leave my bourgeoisie Orange County lifestyle, the kids, my job, and move to Paris, or back to Berlin, and ride the buses."*

I didn't think about *"riding-the-bus"* again until November 2017, when I ran across an excerpt in *Dwelling in the Mirror: A Study of Illusions*, by Burke A. George. He didn't mention her by name, but I'm almost sure it was Suzanne Segal's *"getting-on-the-bus"* experience, from her book, **"Collision with the Infinite:** *A Life Beyond the Personal Self."*

Burke wrote: *"The following is part of a blurb from a best-selling book about a woman's supposed enlightenment: one day over twelve years ago, as a young American woman living in Paris, she stepped onto a city bus and suddenly and unexpectedly found herself egoless, stripped of any sense of a personal self. Struggling for years to make sense of her mental state, she consulted therapist after therapist. Eventually, she turned to spiritual teachers, coming at last to understand that this was the egoless state, the Holy Grail of so many spiritual traditions, that elusive consciousness to which so many aspire."*

Suzanne Segal shows us: *"Over and over again, how people mistake unrelated events and medical conditions that can start a whole chain of events, beginning with miraculous and unexplainable enlightenment."* Then authoring a book about their experience, and as demand grows giving seminars, and finally gaining a devoted following. What they don't understand is that ego-less or enlightenment is not about being a special personified Jesus Christ, the Virgin Mary, the Buddha, or any of the thousand famous masters of the past. What *"did"* or *"do"* they all have in common? They had an experience! Nothing more.

For them, and those in danger of meditation-produced delusions, please realize the goal of meditation is not to attain special states of consciousness, where life's conflicts magically disappear in an aura of enlightenment. **Meditation just *is*,** and we won't give it a name.

Many Minds and Lives are Shattered by ego-meditation-produced delusions, yoga cults, and church sects. Please be cautious exploring the path for mental, emotional, and spiritual well-being, but most of all, stay alert to specialness. Do not mistake *"fool's gold"* of egoic illusions for spiritual illumination. Incorrect meditation perpetuates, or creates trickeries, however appealing they might be. The Kingdom of God is *within*, and if we look out there, there's no chance of finding *"It."*

2. Mindfulness and Meditation

There is consciousness, and then there is the mind. There is no force on this planet that can bring about an end to the mind's mental continuum. But just as consciousness is like the fathomless, deep blue sky, the mind's endless stream of thoughts, like rain clouds, often obscures our true nature. Does that mean that there is no sky? Or that it is a case of a busy mind having to climb Mt. Everest to see the deep blue sky again. There is a simpler approach. Meditation is the *"natural"* solution to let the clouds pass so we can re-connect with our sky like nature of mindfulness and peace of mind. Meditation reduces symptoms of many inflammatory diseases. Paste the link http://bit.ly/2ntTp2E to read the full story. An ounce of meditation is truly worth a pound of medication. In time, but often later than sooner, most herpes sufferers will do the right thing and try to calm their minds, after they've exhausted most other options. Everyone wants to be rid of *"herpes of the flesh,"* few care to give up their Arginine *"pleasures."*

Medication-to-Meditation: part of the Hermes Protocol and practical guide of mindfulness to achieve wellness. Meditation enhances our ability to:

1. Synchronize the body and mind.
2. Overcome habitual behaviors.
3. Relax within discipline, and
4. Face the world with openness, and without fear.

My first responder tendency is to *"figure-it-out."* Surf the internet, read books, and absorb a lexicon of information about whatever crisis is unfolding. I don't want to entirely discount the *"google-information"* approach. It has its place. However, without wisdom and mindfulness, it often creates more tension, rather than alleviating the problem.

Disciplined Meditation might involve each morning and evening, at a specific time and duration. Mindfulness in meditation combines our senses with the mind's attention on any given object. For example, being mindful of the *breath* is a common form of meditation. Following the breath expands consciousness into being fully present in the *"Now"* moment. But mindfulness can be practiced at any time, not only during meditation, to be fully present in any moment, no matter where or what we're doing.

Mindfulness Instead of *"Thinking-a-Mess"*

1. Eases the physical symptoms of herpes outbreaks.
2. Calms the mind and emotions.
3. Improves consciousness.
4. Increases compassion towards oneself and others.
5. Develops a new sense of love, respect, and
6. Acceptance for moving forward.

Instead of Trying to Escape: into another dimension, mindfulness enables us to find shelter in the present moment when overwhelmed with fear and anxiety. With all the turmoil in the world, it can be difficult to appreciate who we are. If we've never developed compassion or kindness toward ourselves, we will seldom experience peace of mind. Persistent herpetic or COVID-19 outbreaks further undermine and complicate our self-worth. Therefore, we project our own fears and confusion onto others.

Instead of Appreciating our lives, even with the *"reptilian predators"* gnawing on our self-confidence, we take our *"whole"* existence for granted, finding it depressing and burdensome. So, we end up doing all sorts of crazy stuff contrary to our own best interest just to cope. Including getting addicted to legal and/or illegal drugs. Yes, it can be helpful to take Genital Herpes seriously, but not disproportionate to the rest of life. Not to where we're constantly complaining about our "woe-is-me" problem. Preferring isolation over companionship and holding resentments against loved ones and acquaintances, finally resorting to a *"bargaining mentality"* with God, yourself, and others. "I'll be good, as long as…."

"Today I accept personal responsibility for uplifting my life." - RH

Justifications, Daydreaming, or Talking about meditation doesn't help. Formal sitting practice does. By meditation we mean something simple:

1. Sitting on a chair or cushion.
2. Assuming good posture.
3. Developing a sense of *"being."*
4. Developing a *"knowing-wisdom."*
5. Knowing that you are in the right place and time.
6. Right here, right now.

Meditation: allows us to disconnect from our discursive stream of thoughts. However, meditation is not about *"not"* thinking. If it were, most meditators would be institutionalized or *la-la*. It's about observing our thoughts, realizing their transparency, being aware of the deep blue sky that includes them.

Pema Chodron: talks about a *"touch-and-go"* approach with a feather. Every time we become aware that we're thinking again, we simply touch our thought "gently" with a feather, and say to ourselves without judgement, *"thinking."* Then letting it go, placing our attention back on the outbreath. Click here http://bit.ly/2Ev9OM8 as Pema Chodron talks you through a mindfulness meditation practice. Does it happen after thirty minutes or your first session? It may not happen after your last session, but gradually you'll wake up feeling different. Most of our lives are filled with brief moments of *"so-called"* peace, after hours on end of worry and frustration. At the mercy of negative thoughts that provoke feelings of fear, doubt, worry, anxiety, depression, and despair.

Like Ravenous Monkeys: when *"stinking-thinking"* gets tired of gnawing on us, for a few moments we feel relief, only to start the vicious *"thinking"* cycle all over again. Meditation can teach us to separate ourselves from discursive *"gnaw"* thinking and put negative forces back where they belong. In Pandora's Box, they can gnaw on herpes.

If you've been to Marineland or Sea-World, you probably stood behind a giant aquarium glass wall, a serene spectator to a plethora of swirling, hustle-and-bustle, *"Star-Wars"* marine life. More awestruck than concerned for your well-being. In time, for moments, that's what it's like looking at your thoughts when meditating. *"Where did that come from?"*

Meditation is not Escape: but a process of self-awakening, versus *medication* the language of the flesh and the ego. Meditation, the Universe's deep blue sky, and prescription into wellness. Instead of coming to meditation with the same *"knowing"* attitude that has prevailed for most of our lives, we come with an atmosphere of openness to discover who we are at our wisest and most confused, but not making a big deal of either. We acknowledge the pain of Genital Herpes, but don't make herpes THE *"pain."* We learn to respect things without putting the magnifying glass over them. Not belittling, but not fueling either.

3. Three Elements of Meditation

Choose a spot away from the hustle and bustle of daily life, where you'll not be disturbed. Meditate early in the morning. Initially, keep your sessions brief, five to ten minutes.

Aspects of meditation:

1. Posture
2. The object of meditation
3. How to deal with your thoughts

Posture: sit upright on a flat surface, either on a cushion or padded folding chair. The feet planted firmly on the ground with an upright back. Try not to tilt to the front, back, or sideways. Feel well balanced. Good posture is important. An upright/straight back is not an artificial posture, but natural. A stiff back is not.

Do not slouch. It makes breathing more difficult. Don't strain by pulling the shoulders up, pushing the chest out. Don't hold the head down, as if bending to something. If sitting on a chair, allow the legs to rest naturally on the floor, hip width apart. Hands resting, palms open, on the thighs. Keep the heart and eyes unlocked, sitting with an open front. Try not to gaze around. Keep the focus slightly downward, about six feet in front of you. Have a sense of belonging and openness. The mouth is accessible, the openness barely visible, just enough to relax the jaw, face, and neck. This also allows the breath to flow naturally. If there is discomfort, make slight adjustments.

Object of Meditation: be mindful of the out-breath. Sit with a good posture. Keep putting the attention on the OUT breath. As you breathe, be fully present. As the out-breath dissolves, the in-breath happens naturally. Then breathe out again, paying more attention on the out-breath. There is a constant going out, flowing in. Again, and again, keep focusing your attention on the out-breath. As the breath dissolves, the in-breath occurs naturally. No need to follow it. Relaxing, letting go, softening outward, keeping a light awareness of the breath as it goes out, again and again.

Working with Our Thoughts: meditation is NOT about NOT thinking. If it were, we'd all get discouraged. When thoughts arise, we simply and gently say to ourselves, *"thinking."* Like a feather touching a soap bubble, say to yourself *"thinking."* Without judgment. Don't say it out-loud. Say it spiritually. Labeling any thoughts with *"thinking"* gives us leverage to come back to the breath. It doesn't matter what thoughts we have, whether we have herpes thoughts, COVID thoughts, negative thoughts, or benevolent thoughts. All are regarded as *"thinking."* Please don't be shocked by your thoughts. Just label them all as simply *"thinking,"* and go back to the breath: *"thinking,"* back to the breath; *"thinking,"* back to the breath.

The *"practice"* of meditation is precise, but simple. It's our posture that enables us to synchronize the mind and body through the breath and the *"feather"* approach to *"thinking."* We're not working with the mind alone but with both our mind and body. When the two perform together and stay within the *"now-moment,"* they are synchronized. A formal practice of meditation will transition into mindfulness in daily life. We start to feel we deserve this earth, and the earth deserves us, with or without Genital Herpes. From being open and honest with ourselves, we become open and honest with others.

E. Inside Outside Review

"The more neurosis, the more wisdom."
-- Author too wise to be known.

The Mind-Body Connection

"Inside Outside" expands and develops into a deeper understanding of how the inside of Meditation affects the outside of Tapping. Be patient as we progress into being Herpes Free. Begin each day with sitting meditation. Start with five minutes watching or listening to Pema Chodron in a guided meditation. In time, YouTube's hand holding will not be necessary, as you sit on your own. From Meditation transition into Tapping http://bit.ly/2nv2bgN (Brad Yates, "Healing").

Harvard Medical School: Psychiatrist Rick Leskowitz, called it *"the most impressive intervention I've encountered in 25 years of work. EFT is on its way to being recognized as the treatment of choice for PTSD, quicker and more effective than anything else, with improvements not typically seen in standard medication or cognitive-behavioral therapy."*

EFT (Emotional Freedom Techniques), or Tapping, has produced remarkable results, but it's still in early childhood. The reader takes complete responsibility for its use. Further, Reinhard Hermes is not a licensed health professional, and offers the information in this book solely as a life coach. Readers are cautioned and advised to consult their physician, psychologist, psychiatrist, or other licensed health care professional before utilizing EFT/Tapping or any information in this book.

PART FIVE: HERMES PROTOCOL

*"The trouble with life isn't that there is no answer,
it's that there are so many."* - Ruth Benedict

The mind is the forerunner to reality. Thinking and doing make it so. If we find ourselves struggling to accept our feelings about Genital Herpes, look to the mind. The ego-mind loves to point, blame, and reward shame with guilt. That doesn't change the reality of the *"human-condition."* Whether we want to accept this or not, suffering is a normal and appropriate response in many situations. Faced with a chronic health issue like Genital Herpes, it's not unusual to suffer. But when it undermines our well-being to the point of despair, it's time. Time to work with our mind to lead us out of darkness, back into the light.

I've learned to trick the ego's illusions, by *"leaning"* into negative emotions instead of pushing them away or ignoring them by shutting down. The pretend *"that's-not-me"* approach never worked. It twisted and turned my emotional life into spells of unsettled anxiety, anger, and fear.

There are exceptions to the mind's fictitious reality. Physical pain, or terminal medical conditions, can advance into grief, depression, and bleak conclusions. But even then, mindfulness meditation and EFT will benefit those terminally ill and dying. Sometimes to the point of *"a peace that passes all understanding."* The Hermes Protocol is designed to relieve the physical symptoms of Genital Herpes and exchange our anxious herpetic-victim-leotards for a peaceful, super-caped mindfulness mantle. Many of us live our life in a constant sequence of recurring problems. As soon as we're finished with herpes, problems in a relationship appear. Then at work and unfriends in *unsocial* media. And on-and-on-and-on it goes in our *"routine I'm not much, but it's all I think about existence."*

Unless We Wake Up: we are born to die under the influence of disturbed attitudes, and negative reflections. No wonder herpes is breaking out in derisive laughter. Although we say we want to be content, and strain to get the *"things"* to make us happy, few seem truly satisfied with their life, herpes or not.

We Seem Unaware: of how we project *"fantasized ways of living onto ourselves and others."* Thank you, social media, television, and the endless marketing *"water-tortures"* we buy in to. Designed to make us feel *"less-than,"* until we go out and buy *"more-than"* we need, just to feel better. By the time we get home we're guilty and annoyed. When things don't work out as expected, such as chronic herpetic lesions, we get even more aggravated. Suffer another outbreak. Get back on our merry-go-round of blaming and condemning to finish our buffet of misery with an extra helping of resentments. To escape these self-inflicted burdens of suffering, we finally surrender. Bend our knees into a meditation cushion, or an EFT chair.

Eckhart Tolle pointed out in his Present Moment Reminder, *"You are not your mind"* http://bit.ly/2BHXXaD, **Wayne Dyer** in his book, *"There's a Spiritual Solution to Every Problem."* http://amzn.to/2BBVJcJ

We can choose to shift our awareness from being a victim, to a *"healing"* observer. It's often a struggle, and we become addicted to our *"woe-is-me"* mindset without realizing it. The only way out is through the mind, meditation, and an awareness of our habitual thought processes.

Meditating and Tapping every morning and night reinforces the body's *"restorative"* powers, opens its meridian channels to a higher, faster recuperative energy. Tapping has never failed to lift my mood, with feelings of awe and respect for the body's healing capacity. Rather than fixating on herpes, and what's wrong, we look for what's right about our health. The reality is we have a compromised immune system, and herpes will most likely not mystically disappear. Through EFT and meditation, we have options to introduce a higher energy Spirit and not turn an outbreak into World War III. Like walking into a dark room, we can turn the light on at any time. Darkness disappears into a light annoyance. Discover the power of turning on the light of life though meditation, Tapping, and Hermes Protocol that turned this author's life into *herpes freedom* since 2017.

Everything is Energy: from the food we eat, to the clothes we wear, the cars we drive, and the sun that sustains our earth's life. The only difference, they're all vibrating at different frequencies. Slower frequencies appear more solid. This is where our physical problems like herpes show up. Faster frequencies such as light, our emotions, and thoughts are less visible. The fastest frequencies are what Wayne Dyer calls *"Spirit."* The difference between physical and spiritual is like the inner and outer world. Yes, they are part of *"One"* world, but *"two unique expressions of being human."*

Everyone is Biologically Unique: some are faster, others slower in their recovery. While doing the Hermes Protocol, please be deliberate and steady. This is not a fifty-yard dash, but a marathon of getting better *one-day-at-a-time*. If you feel overwhelmed, stick your head back under the covers. Start afresh. Try different protocol combinations until you find the ones that work best with your immune system and well-being.

Hermes Protocol depends on a person's:

1. **State of well-being**, special needs, or circumstances.
2. **Financial resources** necessary for protocols and supplements.
3. **Genital Herpes** outbreak frequency and severity.
4. **Available time** to administer and manage protocols.
5. **Desire to learn** more about each protocol and supplement.
6. **Humility** to ask for help when necessary.

Start Here: at the beginning *"It will get better"* in time if you take the time.

Hair Tissue Mineral Analysis (HTMA) determines vitamin and/or mineral deficiencies and level of toxins. Be cautious before starting a supplement regimen prior to your HTMA results. Otherwise, it may compound an already imbalanced profile. Dr. Wilson has an extensive list of approved *"helpers"* to initiate his program.

Reminder, HTMA kits can be ordered through:

www.aurorahealthandnutrition.com, or www.DrLWilson.com

In hindsight, I would start with the *"Banerji"* Homeopathic Protocol after your HTMA, but only if 100% certain that it's Genital Herpes (HSV-2) and not some other infection. Instead, it was my last protocol, but with it, chronic Genital Herpes outbreaks stopped in May 2017. However, I need to qualify my *"outbreak-free"* status. Remember, association does not necessarily mean cause. It could be that my Herpes Free condition has to do with the many protocols prior to undertaking Banerji. These included:

1. Mineral hair analysis,
2. Nutritional balancing diet,
3. High-dose Vitamin C,
4. Vitamins and mineral supplements,
5. Bob Beck Protocol,
6. BHT,
7. MMS or Chlorine Dioxide, and
8. Essential oils.

The decision of which protocols and supplements to use, and in what order, is largely determined by the results of your HTMA analysis. However, no matter what, start today with a healthy diet. Dr. Wilson's Nutritional Balancing Diet http://bit.ly/2rWOH2Q is one example you may want to consider.

Be Cautious: when using homeopathy like the Banerji protocol. *"It's real medicine, not to be taken lightly."* www.JoetteCalabrese.com According to Calabrese, *"It is acceptable to give some things a try on a whim, in the hopes it will make a difference. This is not so with Homeopathy. Instead, I urge my students and readers to be absolutely certain of what they are treating. "If what someone believed was Genital Herpes turned out to be jock itch, some other fungal infection or eczema instead, the Banerji protocol… if used repeatedly, could actually cause the symptoms it was intended to remove. It wouldn't cause herpes but could cause symptoms that might resemble it. That's how Homeopathy works."*

Banerji Protocol for HSV-2
1. **Camphor 200**, one dose for one day only.
2. **Mercurius Solubilis** (or Mercurius vivus) 200c, twice daily.
3. **Arsenicum Album 200c**, twice daily over many months.

I made one modification to the Banjeri dosing process. I placed the pellets in a twelve-ounce (12-oz.) glass of *"distilled"* water the night before and drank its contents the next day. Remember, thirty (30) minutes before or after eating, but best on an empty stomach.

According to Calabrese, *"In some cases, improvement is reported within days, while in others, there's simply a lessening of presenting symptoms. Still, others report that the eruptions continue to occur but are less intense, shorter in duration and the episodes are fewer and far between. The speed and depth of this protocol is dependent on such factors as the amount of suppression from drug use in the past, the immunity of the person, and drugs the sufferer may presently be taking."*

Chapter 13: Day-to-Day

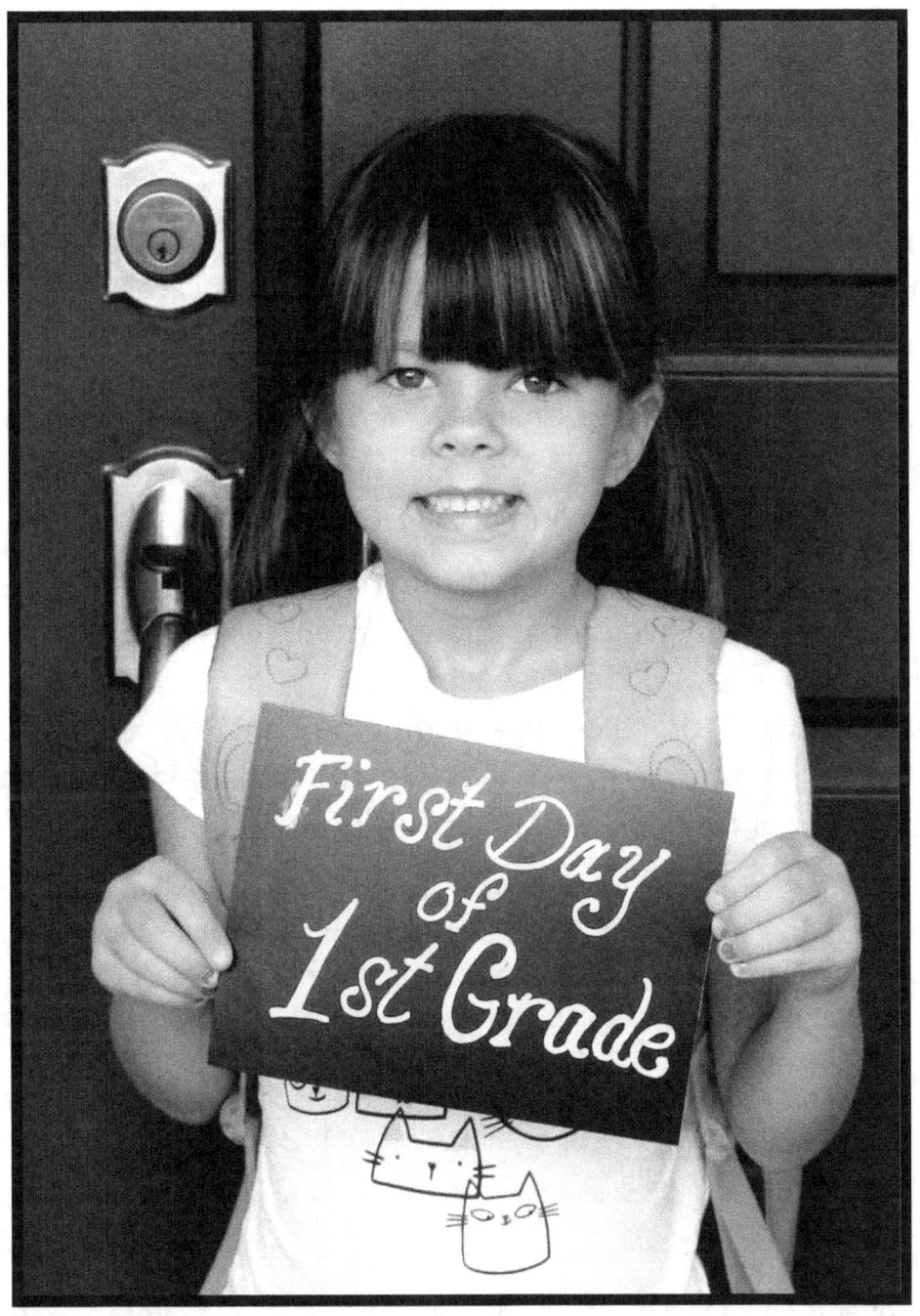

Abigail's First Day as a 1st Grader

A. Morning

*"**Herpes is temporary.** It may last a few hours, a week, a month, or even all year. But eventually it will retreat, go back into hiding, and then something else will take its place. But, if I give up and quit, it will last forever. That concession, a final act of hopelessness, stays with me. So, when I feel like quitting. I ask myself, which would I rather live with?"*

The following supplements, vitamins, hormones, medications, and protocols are an interchangeable combination and part of a morning routine that depends on whether Genital Herpes outbreak(s) are active or not. Remember, the schedule of supplements listed below is a schedule that the author followed at a specific point in time. There are more combinations that may serve your purpose better. Consult with a health care professional about your Hair Mineral Tissue Analysis before starting any protocol.

1. DMSO and MMS

During an active outbreak, after meditating and/or Tapping, but before eating or drinking anything, I applied a *"topical"* blend of DMSO and MMS1 to any active lesions:

Instructions for Topical Application of DMSO and MMS1 to Sacral Herpes:

1. Add five drops un-activated MMS into a one (1) ounce shot-glass.
2. Activate MMS with five drops of four percent (4%) HCL.
3. Wait sixty to ninety (60 to 90) seconds.
4. Then add five (5) drops of one-hundred percent (100%) pure DMSO.
5. Wait two-minutes, add five-to-ten (5 to 10) drops of distilled water.
6. When ready, lightly dab it on to any lesions.

Caution: Add more drops of distilled water for sensitive skin. Also, make sure to test DMSO for sensitivity or allergy first. Put one or two drops inside the forearm, then three or four. Topical DMSO mixture applications and strengths can vary according to past results and experience. Lemon balm or Lysine can also be mixed with DMSO at strengths of 50% to 90% percent, instead of mixing it with MMS1. It's a trial-and-error *"sacral"* process to determine the highest concentration that doesn't cause excessive irritation or reddening of the skin. You can add Aloe Vera gel to make the DMSO cream less harsh. The earlier treatment starts, the better results.

2. Proteolytic Enzymes

Half an hour after taking a teaspoon of DMSO in 2 ounces of Aloe Vera juice and applying a topical mixture of MMS1-DMSO to any active outbreak, I take enzymes and Thyroid Medication. Proteolytic enzyme deficiencies can contribute to herpes outbreaks by affecting your thyroid health. Proteolytic enzymes function as natural immune modulators that can help bring the immune system into balance. http://bit.ly/2EsxQYi

IMPORTANT: unlike *"digestive"* enzymes that are taken with meals to break down food, *"proteolytic"* enzymes are taken *"away"* from food, on an empty stomach. Their purpose is to initiate various chemical reactions within the body. *"The clinical use of enzymes is practiced widely in Germany. They're commonly used for their anti-inflammatory, immune-supportive and blood-thinning properties. Over 50 studies have confirmed their effectiveness in treating rheumatoid arthritis, osteoarthritis, sports injuries, heart health and 'immune function. One systemic oral enzyme is the number one non-aspirin, over-the-counter medicine for pain and inflammation in Germany."* And that's in the country that gave birth to Bayer Aspirin.

Safety and Side Effects: do not take proteolytic enzymes if nursing or pregnant, have a history of ulcers, or taking blood thinners. Also, do NOT take them at least a week before having elective surgery. If in doubt, please contact your health care provider and make certain proteolytic enzymes are appropriate for your health.

3. **Thyroid Medication:** after proteolytic enzymes, I take thyroid medication:
   1. **T-3 Liothyronine** 5 mcg tablet.
   2. **Armour Thyroid** 60 MG.

Thyroid medications are the second top-selling category of drugs in the U.S. According to the American Thyroid Association (ATA) http://bit.ly/2rYGifo an estimated 20 million Americans have some form of thyroid disease. Many of them take Nature-Thyroid, NP Thyroid, or Armour Thyroid, *desiccated, dried thyroid products* made from animal glands. Most are made from a pig's thyroids, replacing, or providing additional thyroid hormones normally produced by our thyroid.

Armour Thyroid: has a long history and is cost effective. Do not supplement with iron, calcium, or aluminum (found in antacids) within four hours of dosing. They interfere with thyroid hormone absorption. In Mexico desiccated thyroid hormones are sold over the counter. They are a prescription in the United States. Most people tolerate them without problems. However, there are exceptions. If a person has a thyroid disorder called thyrotoxicosis, or adrenal gland complications not controlled with treatment, they may not be able to take desiccated thyroid hormones. **Optimizing Thyroid Hormones** is critical for proper immune function. Especially for those who suffer from chronic herpes infections, blood sugar imbalances, sleep disorders, emotional stress, malabsorption issues, or other systemic infections (h-Pylori or dental infections). In short, anything that disrupts the normal state of the body creates hormone imbalances. Until those stressors are dealt with, it is unlikely to experience good health and be *"Herpes-Free."*

Stress causes the body to release cortisol (adrenal hormone) to douse inflammatory fires. If the body is constantly stressed, it will have chronically high cortisol levels, which can cascade into a blood sugar roller-coaster-ride. As a final insult, stress inhibits the conversion of Thyroid T4 to active T3 hormone. *"Goodnight, and welcome to being constantly tired, immune compromised, and never-ending Genital Herpes outbreaks."* Furthermore, decreased T4 to T3 conversion can lower body temperature, dropping immune functions even further, as enzyme efficiency declines. Hormones are like an orchestra. Each member plays an "instrumental" role. But, the conductor (thyroid) and his baton (adrenal cortisol), should be synchronized since they arrange and involve most other hormones. *"Not now, trumpets! Slower, violins. Wake-up, kettlebells."*

Thyroid Hormone T-3: a study published in Cell & Bioscience, March 2017: *"Thyroid hormone (T-3) has been suggested to participate in the regulation of herpesvirus replication during reactivation. Clinical observations and in vivo experiments suggest that T-3 is involved in the suppression of herpes virus replication."* In plain English, optimal T-3, minimal herpes outbreaks. http://bit.ly/2noTMfO

Desiccated Thyroid Hormone: like Armour, contains both T-4 and T-3, but if the body has a T-4 to T-3 conversion issue, or locked cell communication problem, supplementing directly with small doses of T-3 can help significantly. **It works like this**. *"When the body needs energy, it removes an iodine atom from T-4 and turns it into T-3, which then signals cells to make energy (ATP). In other words, T-3 allows the body to turn up the metabolism or energy of the body when it needs it most."* If there is a conversion or signaling issue, not much happens, including not having enough *"oomph"* to get-out of bed and confront *"herpes."*

It's critical to have thyroid hormones in proper balance; otherwise, Genital Herpes outbreaks may only be one of many chronic diseases you experience. In plain English, if the thyroid isn't working right, neither are you. A problem with many orthodox trained doctors is that they focus on thyroid-stimulating hormone, or TSH, and occasionally T4, to determine thyroid health. But TSH and T4 could be normal because the problem is not in the thyroid. It's a conversion issue from T4 to T3 inside the cells. When you mention T-3 to a conventional endocrinologist, they often get a look on their face as if they've just been cornered by T-Rex, instead of T-3.

The pharmaceutical industry has conditioned doctors into believing that T-3 is a voodoo-elixir, and only irrational *"types"* would consider it. Not true. Clinical observations and in vivo experiments suggest that T-3 is involved in the suppression of herpes virus replication. Find an alternative Thyroid practitioner who specializes in endocrinology and is outside mainstream pharmaceutical *"pay-to-play"* rules. A good place to start is at https://stopthethyroidmadness.com/ or The American College for Advancement in

Medicine at www.acam.org. Another option is The American Academy of Anti-Aging Medicine (A4M). They have doctors worldwide dedicated to preventive health.

4. Coconut-Whey-Espresso

Good morning, America! Hello, espresso and coconut oil. While the espresso machine is warming, take a coffee mug, add about one-and-a-half to two (1½ to 2) tablespoons of organic coconut oil, place it on the mug warmer, and wait impatiently until it melts. Then add a tablespoon of *"clean"* Whey Chocolate Protein Isolate, and quarter (1/4) teaspoon of ground Saigon cinnamon. After hand whipping it into a creamy, mellifluous liquid solution, fill the mug with *"espresso-coffee."* Good for some. Trigger for others.

Triggers Common to Many: who suffer from recurrent Genital Herpes outbreaks. These can include **chocolate and caffeine**, but more often it's a lack of sleep, menstruation, colds/flu, illnesses, and pretty much anything else that compromises the immune system.

Caffeine can affect herpes by stimulating the adrenal glands to produce adrenalin, the *"flight or fight"* hormone that jolts us. Now imagine the body being in retreat or conflict *"mode"* all day, every week, for the entire year. What do you suppose are the effects on the adrenals? A constant state of stress depletes them, even if we're just sitting at our desk sipping a morning cup of java. Caffeine is a stimulant, neither good nor bad. But like any drug, the more we take, the more resistant the body becomes. One cup in the morning can gradually lead to two or three (2 or 3) to get the same response. It's not long before the immune system is negatively impacted, allowing herpes to gain the upper hand.

Whether caffeine induces herpes outbreaks depends on the oral intake, adrenalin secreted, and impact on the immune system. Read, *Caffeine And Herpes: Good And Bad* http://bit.ly/2BJq6hC.

There is a growing body of literature that suggests that moderate coffee consumption brings health benefits besides its morning pick-me-up. According to the Mayo Clinic and Medical News Today, it strengthens heart and liver health and reduces the risk of certain cancers. Consuming at least 2 cups a day can also boost cognitive function, reduce the risk of Alzheimer's disease, and improve a person's writing ability. Sorry, I'm hoping this next cup will help. The unwelcome news for caffeine junkies, consuming more than three or four cups per day, its benefits decline.

B. Lunch

1. Supplements and Budwig Diet

Lunch is the biggest meal of the day. Besides digestive enzymes, I take most of my vitamins and minerals according to the Hair Tissue Mineral Analysis . Two or three times a week I eat *"The Budwig Diet,"* with two cups of steamed vegetables.

Dr. Johanna Budwig: (1908-2003) a German biochemist, was a seven-time Nobel Prize nominee, and a world-renowned physicist and pharmacist. Dr. Budwig was a persuasive advocate for consuming flax seed oil (The Budwig Protocol) to cure many metabolic diseases. She scientifically connected the relationship between cancer research and fat metabolism. www.budwigcenter.com

Based on her extensive scientific research, Dr. Budwig developed a diet that proved successful in treating many metabolic diseases, but specifically cancer. She had an unheard-of success rate, similar to Dr. Max Gerson. Unlike in the U.S., where most successful alternative cancer clinics have been shut down by the FDA, they continue to flourish in Europe and South America, many still staunch advocates of her cancer diet. **The Budwig Diet** emphasizes healthy fats, high antioxidant fresh vegetables, fermented probiotic rich dairy products, sauerkraut, cottage cheese, organic yogurt, flaxseeds, and flaxseed oil. The diet is referred to as the Flaxseed Oil Diet. Today, Dr. Mercola has continued Dr. Budwig's mission to educate the public on why healthy dietary fat is crucial http://bit.ly/2GBoZnP.

2. Apple Cider Vinegar (ACV)

ACV helps the immune system alkalize the body, kill candida, and keep Genital Herpes under control. For lunch add two tablespoons of ACV into a 16 oz. empty glass bottle, then mix in a quarter teaspoon of baking soda. Wait until the fizzing stops, and fill with clean, pure water. Drink half during lunch and the other half with dinner. ACV strengthens the gut flora and body's immune system, which will help keep the herpes virus dormant. Start with one or two (1-or-2) teaspoons in a glass of water and increase the amount slowly. While ACV works well for most people, some experience side effects. Start slow and increase the dosage gradually. http://bit.ly/2EsUG1X

3. Banerji Protocol: take before or after lunch

1. **Mercurius Solubilis** (or Mercurius Vivus) 200c, twice daily.
2. **Arsenicum Album 200c,** twice daily over many months.

Banerji Dosing Process: take the pellets 30 minutes before or after eating, but it's best on an empty stomach.

C. Dinner & Evenings

Before retiring for the evening, I take two supplements and three medications to boost the immune system in its battle against Genital Herpes and infections:

1. Proteolytic Enzymes
2. DMSO (During an Outbreak)
3. Nature-Thyroid
4. Liothyronine (T-3 Thyroid Hormone)
5. Melatonin
6. LDN (Low Dose Naltrexone)

DMSO and MMS

Repeat the morning procedure during an active outbreak. Take one teaspoon of 99.9% pharmaceutical grade DMSO in two ounces of Aloe Vera juice. Apply a "topical" blend of DMSO and MMS1 to any active lesions:

Mixture Instructions for Topical Application of DMSO and MMS1 to Sacral Herpes Lesions:

1. **Add 5 drops** of un-activated MMS into a one ounce (1) shot-glass.
2. **Activate MMS** using five (5) drops of 4% HCL, wait 60 seconds.
3. **Add** five to seven (5 to 7) drops of 100% DMSO.
4. **Wait 2 minutes,** then add five to ten (5 to 10) drops of distilled water.
5. **When ready,** lightly dab on any lesions.

Proteolytic Enzymes

Dosage: After the first week, take one capsule in the morning, one at night, preferably two or three (2 or 3) hours after dinner:

1. **Keep the dosage** at two (2) capsules for the next week.

2. **If there is no discomfort,** increase to three (3) capsules a day, in any combination, both in the morning and at night. For example, take two capsules AM and one PM.

3. **For most,** two to three (2-3) capsules a day is an optimum long-term dose. However, for those suffering from debilitating and chronic inflammation, consider taking one full dose in the morning, another in the evening.

Armour-Thyroid and T-3

After lunch (2:00 pm) but before dinner, take sixty (60) mg of Armour Thyroid and five (5) mcg of T-3. It's been my experience that thyroid meds are better absorbed if enzymes are taken first. Please make sure NOT to take any calcium or iron supplements at least three or four (3 or 4) hours before or after taking your thyroid medication.

Melatonin

Melatonin Regulates the body's internal clock, the sleep cycle. But it carries out a *"vast array of other tasks,"* including regulating certain immune responses (herpes), protecting the body against radiation exposure, and tinnitus. Melatonin supplements cause few side effects but can interact with (Rx) pharmaceutical drugs. Talk with your pharmacist or health care provider if you're taking any medication to make certain melatonin will not interfere and cause unwanted side effects.

I found an interesting small study, *"Regression of herpes viral infection symptoms using melatonin and SB-73 in comparison with Acyclovir."* http://bit.ly/2FxldKX *"The aim of the study was to investigate if 2.5 mg melatonin and 100 mg SB-73 would help patients with herpes, and to compare it to a control group who took 200 mg Acyclovir. SB-73 is a mixture of magnesium, phosphate, fatty acids extracted from Aspergillus, which has anti-herpes virus properties. Almost 96% of the melatonin patients reported a complete regression of symptoms after seven (7) days of treatment. By comparison, 85.3% of the Acyclovir group reported regression of symptoms in the same period. There was a statistically significant difference between the groups."* A ten percent difference may not seem much, but we're talking Acyclovir, orthodox medicine's standard-of-care for all herpes infections, versus two-and-a-half (2.5) mg of melatonin and a few vitamins. But we'll never read about it in *The Times* or hear it on CNN.

Jeff T. Bowles, <u>Extreme Dose! Melatonin,</u> the *Miracle Anti-Aging Hormone* is a valuable resource to learn more about Melatonin's benefits. Bowles has been known to take substantial amounts up to five-hundred milligrams (500 mg) without side effects, other than sleeping fourteen (14) hours a day. http://amzn.to/2DUmmQg Books by Bowles.

Dosage: I've taken three mg to as much as 50 mg a night, but never more than waking up refreshed. If you are groggy and sleepy in the morning after taking melatonin, it may be too large a dose. Build up slowly. My last supplement before going to bed is **melatonin.** Like MMS, Vitamin C, and T-3, there are a lot of melatonin warnings and misinformation about consuming more than 3 mg. Read Jeff Bowles book on **Melatonin**. He has the research and personal clinical experience to offer more than biased propaganda. In Europe, melatonin is used as an adjunct for birth control at a dose of 75 mg a night. http://wapo.st/2nskCnf

LDN (Low Dose Naltrexone)

LDN is an *"off-label"* medication approved by the FDA and used frequently by "alternative" doctors to treat autoimmune diseases. Taken at bedtime, LDN works by briefly blocking opiate receptors and *"tricking"* the body into increasing endorphin production. Endorphins are a vital part of a healthy immune system that LDN facilitates to correct immune defects.

Bernard Bihari, MD, discovered the clinical effects of LDN in humans with his 1985-86 groundbreaking clinical trial with HIV/AIDS patients. Dr. Bihari realized the effectiveness of LDN in protecting an HIV battered immune system. In some of Bernard Bihari's earliest studies, he applied the same HIV/AIDS principles of LDN to the treatment for herpes. http://bit.ly/2s4Gjyz One of Bihari's first patent applications was for the use of LDN in HIV herpes infections. Elaine A. Moore, *"The Promise of Low Dose Naltrexone Therapy,"* is credible up-to-date information about Low Dose Naltrexone (LDN) for patients, physicians, and researchers that can be found at www.LDNScience.org.

Dose and Frequency: begin with three (3.0) mg per day and adjust the dosage if necessary. Prescribing one-and-a-half (1.5) mg capsules allows for easy adjustment. For example, a client can take either two capsules for three (3) mg, or three capsules for a four-and-a-half (4.5) mg dose.

Side Effects: some patients report vivid dreams, others occasionally complain of difficulty sleeping. If this persists after the first week, dosage can be reduced from four-and-a-half (4.5) mg to three (3) mg. LDN is essentially non-toxic, simple to administer, and inexpensive, $90 per month.

D. Detoxification

Instead of Being in Conflict: let Genital Herpes motivate us to untangle and transform our perceptions of life's disappointments. That way we'll be prepared to face those in the future. Genital Herpes is like a sword, frequently wounding and scarring relationships, and cutting through our illusions. As we look at our life, as it represents itself in our hearts, can we accept the truth? To live with or without herpes is to experience pain, joy, sorrow, happiness, loss, and grief. It's all part of the human condition that we all have in common.

A bigger problem than herpes is for those who can't see or feel that. Unintentionally making them in constant conflict with life itself. Just as sadness can be the wellspring of creativity, happiness a fountain of authenticity, let herpes be the motivator for peace of mind. Some of us get anxious every time we feel that *"tingling"* sensation of an imminent outbreak. Others simply go about their day. Physiologically the way herpes initially interacts within each person's ecology is much the same.

Depending on an individual's immune system, the stages of herpes take on a standard sequence. But here's where it gets interesting. The anxious person takes the long way home, stopping at CVS to pick-up her script of Acyclovir. Still, it takes three (3) weeks for remission and healing.

The *"go about their day"* person doesn't bother with antivirals and still the infection disappears within ten (10) days. There is not much we can do about our biological or innate immunity. It exists by virtue of a person's genetic make-up. The difference, and just as important, is our subconscious beliefs, and state-of-mind.

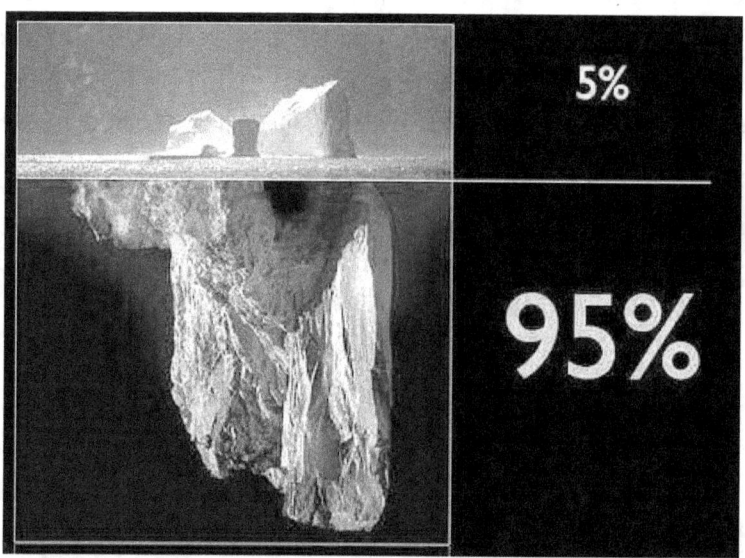

The Conscious Mind: only controls the brain five-percent (5%) of the time. I thought, *"No way!"* My mind is like a jumping flea. Giving it five-percent (5%) was kind. I'm kidding, but it's certainly believable that the subconscious has a hold of our thoughts 95% of the time. http://bit.ly/2DRm5K0

Even if the conscious mind thinks, *'I am healthy,'* the subconscious mind may be running a different database and a more powerful program in the background. Such as 'I have bad genes and my family has a history of cancer.' Genes are merely a blueprint to health, while the mind is responsible for interpreting that plan. It's up to us to decide how we want our health proposal to manifest. How do we do that?

By managing our thoughts and emotions. When your thoughts are negative, fear-based, or stress-induced, the body responds by turning off the immune system. But if our conscious and subconscious mind are aligned with positive thoughts, the body responds with enhanced healing and health. Thoughts are real. They have a biological and physiological effect. The body responds to mental input as if it was a physical reality. So, how do we change our subconscious beliefs? We detoxify the mind through *Tapping and meditation*.

Detoxify or Acidify

It's important to wash your car before detailing it. Emptying the trash before replacing it with a new liner. Taking off soiled sheets before putting on clean ones. Showering after a workout before stepping into clean underwear. And *not over-supplementing in advance of detoxifying;* otherwise, all desired outcomes can be contaminated.

The ER physician first stops the bleeding, just as the Hermes Protocol aims to improve chronic Genital Herpes infections. Our goal is to leave the ER of our own accord. To have the immune system keep us outbreak free without our constant intervention. So, take the trash out, and reestablish immunity.

Today, everyone, including newborn babies are toxic and mineral deficient. It's disturbing to find more than 200 chemicals in African American, Hispanic, and Asian newborns. *"The study focused on minority children to show that chemical exposure is ubiquitous. Building on 2005 research on cord blood taken from ten anonymous babies."* http://bit.ly/2rYX8e6

Toxins that Distress the Body:

1. **Toxic chemicals,** from pesticides and insecticides, food additives, packaging materials, factory pollutants, car exhaust, building materials, etc.

2. **Biological toxins** called endotoxins and exotoxins, secreted from viruses (like herpes), bacteria, parasites, and fungi. Another source of biological toxins is the use of vaccines, booster shots, and flu shots. They not only introduce the intended virus or germ, but many are contaminated with other viruses, chemicals, and toxic metals.

3. **Mental and emotional toxins** created by our *"mind's"* negative attitude toward Genital Herpes, and ensuing harmful ideas, false beliefs, unreal perspectives, which can lead to depression and/or anxiety.

4. **Trauma** of all kinds, including physical (herpes infections), mental, and/or emotional, can cause severe dysfunction in the body and mind.

5. **Electrical and electromagnetic** toxins from cell phones, 220-volt wiring, TV sets, computer screens, high-tension power lines, transformers, junction boxes, fluorescent light, and many more. Hello, cell phones, goodbye bees, adios pollination, and where have all the fruits and veggies gone?

6. **Industrialization,** over-use of plastics and careless use of toxic chemicals, has combined to contaminate our air, food, and water supply. In addition to the traditional pollutants, we are now faced with a more insidious and newer hazard that may be worse. Utilities across the country are installing so-called 'smart' meters.

7. **Wireless,** not only are electrical bills skyrocketing, but their health effects and safety concerns have shot up dramatically. Do we really need wireless smart meters? I mean, are we that dumb to believe that the same technology in cell phones that causes brain

tumors, now magnified by a gazillion, is somehow OK in our homes? Once installed, frequently there is no right to opt out. Thousands upon thousands of people have complained of tinnitus, headaches, nausea, sleeplessness, heart arrhythmia, and many other symptoms after these *'stupid'* smart meters were installed.

IMPORTANT: Wireless technology is a physical health hazard. Its addictive use is a precursor to mental infertility and emotional immaturity.

Like Cancer Rates: electromagnetic pollution is getting worse, not better. To the point that today everyone is toxic. It only comes down to how heavy a load. **Newsflash:** toxins cause untold suffering and sickness, the cruelest of which is malignancy. People who feel tired all the time may just be carrying a heavy toxic load. Like driving an overloaded dump truck with a burned-out dashboard and the emergency brake on.

You keep glaring at the *"smart"* speedometer, wondering what's wrong. But no matter what you do, you limp along, worn out, with creaks and cranks escaping from an overburdened and weakened frame. Your dashboard is blank, and health "specialists" think it's all in your head. They suggest maybe you should get a change of scenery or therapy. An *impolite* way of saying, you're *"depressed."* The last *"specialist"* who looked at your labs did mention that your liver enzymes were slightly elevated, although she didn't seem that concerned. *"It's nothing to worry about. Cut back on red meat."*

Most Rx Lab Values: are like automobile dashboards. They don't tell you anything unless something is already broken. Otherwise, why do we see so many stranded, overheated cars, hooked up to a tow-truck? They started okay that morning. Their *"smart-dashboard"* said, *"All is well,"* even though it wasn't. When your doctor looks at your labs, they see a *"normal"* reference range, taken from overweight, toxic, unhealthy people, who were advised to do bloodwork.

Normal Ranges are calculated: so that 95% of *"healthy"* people have values that fall within the normal range. The catch-22 is the word *"healthy."* We all know how healthy most people are. If you want to be like them, then let the *"all-is-well"* lab values be your guide. But if you want to cruise through life like a well-maintained F-150, maintain a healthy lifestyle and diet, with appropriate supplements. Drop the toxic load you've been hauling around at the nearest dump and change the oil with a yearly detoxification protocol.

Detox. Your liver and kidneys will reward you with better health. It may be what the *"immune system"* needs to motivate Genital Herpes to crawl back into its cave. To be human and live an active life, there's not much we can do to avoid these ubiquitous toxins. These simple suggestions may help. First, minimize chemical exposure with a nutrient rich, organic diet. Drink plenty of purified water. Use natural household products and cosmetics. Don't use pesticides or herbicides to make that lawn or your plants *"look"* greener. If you jog or ride a bike, avoid heavy traffic. If all else fails, move to Alaska.

Eliminate toxins: from the body. But like any battlefield, if the *"good guys"* are endlessly engaged trying to suppress one infection after another, it'll only be a matter of time before immunity weakens and eventually succumbs. When that happens, our weakened immune system can get confused and mistake the good guys for the bad. With crippled resistance, confused, unable to do its job, the immune system strikes out in all directions, attacking its own, and eventually succumbing to some opportunistic disease. In an odd way, we can be grateful for herpes playing *"the"* canary in a mineshaft. It's warning us to shore up our defenses and strengthen the immune system. The best support we can give our body is to stop adding more toxins, eliminate those already stored in our system.

Supplements and procedures that may help:

1. **Detoxify the Liver.** It's the first and most important organ of detoxification, followed by the kidneys and our skin. There are several first-rate liver protocols but start by improving your diet. Then take some extra supplements to help detoxify.

2. **Eat Cruciferous Vegetables.** Even though they're goitrogenic and a problem for some hypothyroid individuals, they support healthy liver function and detoxification. If you're hypothyroid but iodine sufficient, normal amounts shouldn't be a problem.

3. **Eat Garlic.** Allicin in garlic helps detoxify the liver. A side benefit it also keeps Genital Herpes in check.

4. **Cilantro** may help remove heavy metals and is commonly included in certain detoxification products.

5. **Chlorella** is often called a super-food and may help remove heavy metals such as cadmium and mercury. It can prevent the accumulation of dioxins within the body.

6. **Milk Thistle** is one of the most popular herbs to protect and improve liver health. It may even prevent the formation of gallstones. Silymarin is the active ingredient.

7. **Globe Artichoke** is an herb that is useful for liver toxicity or damage. It can also help improve bile production.

8. **Dandelion** is another herb to help to improve liver function.

9. **Schisandra** is an antioxidant berry to improve the detoxifying capacity of the liver, both for acute and chronic liver diseases.

10. **Infrared sauna therapy** is beneficial in eliminating toxins, improving circulation, and reducing blood pressure. Many healthcare professionals recommend using sauna therapy, including Dr. Mark Hyman, Dr. Joseph Mercola, and Dr. Lawrence Wilson. Some endorse *infrared saunas*; others favor **far** *infrared sauna*. Both are beneficial. Most units sold are *far infrared saunas*.

11. **CAUTION:** many herpes sufferers have a love-hate relationship with the sun, sweating, and sweltering heat. If Genital Herpes breaks out with every fever, day at the

beach, or from sweating every time you work out, skip the sauna until the predator is back in its box.

12. **Activated Charcoal** is made from bone char, coconut shells, peat, or sawdust. Its medical use dates to Hippocrates (400 B.C.) when physicians treated epilepsy and anthrax with it. After the development of the charcoal activation process (1870 to 1920), reports appeared in medical journals about its use as an antidote for poisons and intestinal disorders. Porous and negatively charged, it helps bind a variety of toxins, preventing them from being absorbed into the body.

Activated charcoal is ordinarily considered safe, but for some it can cause unpleasant gastro-intestinal side effects. If you have any medical conditions such as intestinal bleeding or blockages, recent abdominal surgery, activated charcoal may not be for you. Check with your doctor. Activated charcoal can also interfere with the absorption of nutrients, supplements, and prescription medications. Take activated charcoal 90 minutes to two hours prior to meals, supplements, and medications. Always check with your health-care provider if these conditions apply before taking activated charcoal.

Cleanse the Colon

There are numerous ways to clean the colon. If you go online, or walk into any local health food store, there is no shortage of kits or supplements to cleanse the colon.

Coffee Enemas: Dr. Max Gerson's promoted coffee enemas to detoxify the liver, increase glutathione production, and eliminate pathogens. As a side benefit they cleanse the colon. The other advantages of coffee enemas? They are done in the privacy of your home and are cost effective.

My initial reaction at a Max Gerson seminar www.Gerson.org was, *"What?"* Sorry, but I take my macchiato espresso through the esophageal tube, not my sphincter. Despite my initial suspicion, by the time I finished the seminar and looked at the science, I decided to try them. It took a while to overcome the mental resistance. But the first time I heard that all familiar gallbladder *"squirt,"* and my temperature went back to normal, I quickly saw their benefit. Dr. Wilson's website has complete details on how to go about taking a coffee enema. http://bit.ly/2BKgsv9

Colon hydrotherapy and colonic irrigation are other methods to clean the colon. For colon hydrotherapy/colonic irrigation it's best to see a certified hydro-therapist. The advantage of colon hydrotherapy is that it does a better job of cleansing when compared to coffee enemas. However, for some people, it is too aggressive. If you have intestinal permeability (a leaky gut), it's best to refrain from colon hydrotherapy.

Whatever method(s) you decide to use, consider a liver-kidney-colon detox program to support the immune system in its efforts to keep Genital Herpes dormant. Finally, detoxification is not a 100-yard dash, but a New York marathon. Start all doses and protocols low and slow. Work your way up. Try not to do too much all at once. Detoxing will take anywhere from thirty (30) days to several months. Sometimes longer. Also, pulse your treatments on and off. Otherwise, they'll lose their effectiveness.

Water Advice: don't underestimate the importance of drinking and using purified water in your home. The worst offender is fluoride. Unlike chlorine, fluoride is not eliminated by boiling water. The best solution is to install a kitchen sink and shower filter that removes fluoride or purchase bottled water but make sure they contains no toxic chemicals.

Clipping Corners

Knowledge is power, but excessive knowledge is weakness. If you decide to use the Hermes Protocol (HP), do your research. Well-informed advocates make better choices. Once you decide, stay the course until you're Herpes Free.

The Hermes Protocol can be intensive, expensive, and overwhelming because of its lifestyle changes, supplements, treatments, and mind-therapies. But as Thomas Jefferson wrote, *"The price of freedom is eternal vigilance."* Well, so is the price of *Herpes Freedom*. If you falter, pick yourself back up. Brush off the temptation to quit before the miracle happens. Get back on the diet, adjust your supplements, meditate, and trust your inner voice. If you're still uncertain, ask for help. *From Genital Herpes to the Hermes Protocol, into Herpes Freedom.*

Chapter 14: In Closing

*"Herpes is temporary. But if I give up and quit,
those feelings will last forever. Which would I rather liver with?"* - RH

It is my sincere hope that you have found solace and relief with the Hermes Protocol. Remember, it was *"key"* that let *darkness* out from Pandora's box? So, it's *key* for us to purify the body and purge the mind of gloom. Unlocking the body-mind connection, as we let go of our negative emotions. Thank you for your efforts in looking for a solution, rather than a quick fix.

I believe the Hermes Protocol's mental approach to physical health challenges will benefit any situation. If you have questions or concerns, please feel free to contact me at rhermes1@gmail.com, and I will respond to you as quickly as I can. Now for a few final observations. No matter what our current life's circumstance, or what we've done, or *"they"* did. If we allow ourselves to be dominated by herpes outbreaks, their negative emotions, and undesirable thoughts, we will experience a continuous cycle of infections, problems, confusion, and loneliness.

Healing the burden: Genital Herpes does not occur through blame or judgement, or by being in denial. It's the willingness to discern without judgement. To see life as it is, so we can live openly in truth, no matter what. Eventually, we come to realize that **"My Friend, the Enemy,"** is not only herpes, but many times the person looking back at us from the mirror.

People who have gone through personal tragedies, the loss of a loved one, divorce, cancer, combat, or PTSD, say that what got them through was thinking back to a time when someone loved them unconditionally. Whether it was their wife, lover, Mom or Dad, or an uncle, who loved them without conditions. Even if it was only for a moment. Yes, inside that space of time they knew love and felt lovable. It doesn't take much, just one person in one moment. Maybe it's time to extend that mercy to ourselves while undertaking the Hermes Protocol. Everyone carries a certain amount of cosmic pain that the Universe entrusts. Those with chronic herpes bear an extra serving. Yet, when called upon to endure it, we do so with acceptance. Not self-pity. It's part of our human condition.

It's time to get over the fixed idea, *"My life should be a certain way, especially without herpes."* Remember, we don't control life's ingredients, only what we do with them. So, no matter what physical or mental problems we experience, instead of getting anxious and fearful, sit back, relax, be as still as possible. See their reality and face the solution to be Genital Herpes FREE. Try to understand the virus through our wisdom, not fear. Realize, most of our difficulties will fade in time, or just disappear. It's Life.

A. Peace for Happiness

Is it fair to tell someone who's going through a challenging time in their marriage, a demanding supervisor, chronic herpes infections, or a monetary crisis to just *"change your attitude and everything will be OK?"* On a simplistic level that's what many therapies champion. I've heard the trite advice, *"Just get it together, and stop complaining. Get over it."* Just because your wife is leaving you, your son is in prison, or you have cancer, is no reason to always be so gloomy. Do something about it. Either change yourself or the situation. Find some happiness. *"Run, Forrest! Run!"* As quickly as you can, get away from such insensitive rubbish.

Genital Herpes Question Remains: can we be happy with chronic herpes infections? Or is there something inherently wrong with the way we live? No matter what happens or what we do, there are always going to be problems, sadness, and pain. Even after outbreaks stop. What's the solution? You're not going to like the answer, but in time you may come to understand what is meant by it.

The Answer: there is no solution. But within that contradiction rests peace and happiness. Know that there is no happiness in this world. What?? You got to be kidding! *"I've read this far, and you're telling I'm going to be miserable for the rest of my life, no matter what?"* Let me explain the wisdom that's buried inside that inconsistency. You have Genital Herpes. That's an imperfection in our immune system and health. Logic says I should be able to find a solution to eliminate outbreaks and be Herpes Free. The relationship with our body is not much different than we have with our spouse, other people, and most things in life. Let's say we're talking about our spouse. My ego tells me I should be able to find a wife or husband who's there for me, who entertains me, but when I want to be left alone, they give me space. Someone who satisfies me, understands my struggles with Genital Herpes.

Bad news. You don't want a partner that's a human being; you want an iPad. Someone that entertains you and makes you laugh, but that you can turn off, and *yet at the ready* when you need them. And if something goes wrong, you just buy the new model. Faster, better, but not cheaper. The problem with replacing your husband, or wife, with a newer model. You'll still be suffering. Because no matter what you do, you'll either have married-person suffering, or single-person suffering. So, it is with Genital Herpes. I've been herpes free since May 2017, but I still experience pain. I've just replaced herpes suffering with _____. What's profound about that experience is that I've been under the delusion that if I could just change the situation for a better one, then I would stop suffering. If only I could have changed my x-wife. Made her see the world according to *"me,"* so her idiosyncrasies wouldn't irritate or annoy me. If she'd only been more loving, then I would've been happy. Or, if I got a better job, or if Golden State wins tonight, or if *blah, blah…* then I would be happy.

The only thing that ever changed was one form of suffering for another. I'm now financially in a demanding situation. So, I'm hoping to win the lotto. But guess what? After reading all the tragedies and how miserable people were after winning the lotto, I realized that I'd just be replacing a **poor-person** with **rich-person** suffering. Reading tabloids headlines confirms that being rich and famous does nothing to eliminate suffering. It may even enhance its effect. Fame and wealth have inherent shortcomings. The only peace I ever found was in the *"now"* moment by being present *"here and now."*

Politicians lure us into believing that if we only had equitable income distribution. Better schools for our children, clean water, and universal prosperity. But guess what? We would still find that there would be universal suffering. I was under the ***"if only"*** **delusion** most of my life. The following cosmopolitan wish list attests to our collective illusions:

1. **If only** I had a better partner in life, so we could live in harmony.
2. **If only** I had the right amount of income, then we'd live comfortably.
3. **If only** I had more considerate children.
4. **If only** I didn't have chronic **Genital Herpes**, then I would be happy.

"Ooops, sorry." I almost forgot. I don't have chronic herpes anymore. I've replaced herpes suffering with publishing distress. Here are other traps. Looking for the imperfection in situations; finding the enemy in others; frequently craving validation; comparing and competing; conditional love; trying to change someone; or fear-projecting the future.

There is no perfect life. It doesn't exist. Halfway through my Herpes Free journey and while drafting this book, I realized there is nothing wrong with me. Not with my brain, or my education. Or even with my body's herpetic eczema history. Pain and suffering are just part of the human condition. There is no getting around being human. It includes failed marriages, children that don't call, bills past due, loneliness, Genital Herpes, and uncertainty about the future. Accepting the pain and grief of divorce is to be at peace with life as it unfolds. My New Year's wish was less than acceptance. *"Please God, don't make this another character-building year."*

Regarding the anguish that can occur in Genital Herpes relationships, it's normal. Everyone I've ever known has been sick at one time or another, with many catching terrible colds or the flu every year. But we don't think of being sick as normal. We see it as something *"wrong"* with us. The only people I know that never get sick are dead. You could call that the ultimate or final illness. By rejecting our sickness as "wrong-ness," we're in denial against the very nature of life. Sickness is part of life and denying and rejecting it is going against the life force.

Acceptance: is the key to healing and transformation. Acknowledging that chronic Genital Herpes can be a common occurrence for a compromised immune system. That there is nothing inherently *"wrong"* with us is the first step in the healing process. What it does to herpes or any disease, it takes away the guilt and shame that surrounds it.

Often, we don't see a doctor because we think there is something immoral or *"wrong"* being infected with Genital Herpes. However, accepting the state of our body, including Genital Herpes, is to be proactive instead of inactive and wishful. Embracing our sickness, whether herpes or any other disease, changes our entire emotional construct into a more peaceful state of mind. Make peace with your herpes history. Our biggest spiritual growth takes place on the back of difficult burdens. Take hold of herpes, even if you need help, turn it into just another hurdle, ingredient in your life's journey.

Embrace the truth and reality of life instead of pushing it away. In acceptance we find a sense of ease, and understanding that we may never have a perfect, healthy body, and the one we have is good enough. With that approach we engage our body instead of rejecting it. With engagement comes a feeling of peace. You begin to realize that we don't have to change who we are. When you accept and honor your history the *"enemy"* will often retire gracefully. Accept all chapters of your life's story, including herpes.

Instead of listening to our faultfinding mind, with its constant selection of negative thoughts spotlighting our defects and those of others, we focus on our appreciative attitudes that embrace our faults and character defects of others. With acceptance something else happens. Often our health improves. Outbreaks are diminished as we acknowledge the pain of Genital Herpes, instead of trying to reject it.

It's the Negativity: we attach to our herpes experience that's the real problem. The lack of tolerance creates more tension, stress, guilt, and pain. The endless desire to escape herpes, wishing things were different, that only causes more suffering. If we accept our condition, part of the disease and stress is removed. Even though antivirals often alleviate outbreaks entirely, it's the mind and our thinking that respond to acceptance and love. Not Valtrex. Stop making herpes the enemy. Embrace and make peace with it, and in the process, free yourself.

For those who meditate, you know the more you try to control the mind and your thoughts, the more problematic the practice becomes. We never get still in meditation by trying to be still. The way to stillness in meditation is to care for the mind with the same compassion and love we tend to our children. In meditation we stop arguing with ourselves, our mind, or our heart. We make peace with every moment. *The real source of happiness is inner peace.* If the mind is peaceful, we are content. So, it's not either peace or happiness, but both inner peace and outer happiness.

B. Fear to Confidence

"I've learned over the years that when one's mind is made up, this diminishes fear; knowing what must be done, does away with fear." - Rosa Parks

Experience Peace and Happiness: transcend fear into confidence. Fear takes many forms with Genital Herpes: from the shock and panic when we first test positive, to the emotional challenges that confront our relationships.

We use countless strategies to take our mind away from or off herpes. Some drink, others do drugs. A few meditate and practice yoga. Many seek refuge in TV or bury themselves in romantic novellas. The adventurous type go to a local pub and have a few beers. Anything not to be alone with our anxious mind. But eventually some of us get fed up with the repetitive routines and boredom sets in. With boredom we are closer to fear. When we're aware of our anxiety, nervousness, and restlessness, it's the beginning of moving beyond them. Underneath fear's glossy veneer, we realize it's nothing more than a smokescreen to protect us from sorrow.

Slow down, Relax, Let Your Guard Down: experience the sadness. A sorrow of the heart. We feel lonely, wishing that herpes hadn't interfered in our life. This is another step toward confidence. If we hide from the world, we may feel more secure and think we've quieted our anxiety, but all we've done is make ourselves numb. Surrounded with our habitual thoughts, hoping nothing else will harm us. We have walled off our hearts. But gradually we come to realize that maybe herpes isn't the enemy. It's our negative stinking thinking. Perhaps if we start to make friends with ourselves by being more human, temperate, and open, we can change. Not into a feeble, milk-and-honey gentleness, but your basic goodness kind, from which we gain strength and confidence. Confidence that doesn't come about through self-improvement but in aligning our body and mind to thrive in concert. In their harmony we alleviate our fears.

The body can be compared to the camera in your iPhone. The mind is the memory chip. The question is how to use them together to get a clear, accurate picture of our world. Only if the aperture, shutter speed, and memory chip are aligned, can we take accurate images. Similarly, when the mind and body are properly synchronized we get a more accurate, unblemished vision of our world. Without blurry shortsightedness, we begin to trust ourselves and have less anxiety.

Instead of Being Ashamed: in who we are, our job, finances, relationships, education, and our mental shortcomings, we begin to synchronize the mind and body to connect to the world with confidence. This process affects how we see ourselves. We begin to form a more accurate perception of Genital Herpes, and that no matter what, we have a perfect right to be in this world, just as we are.

We look, we see, and we know. Most of all, we don't apologize for being. As we experience the honesty of being alive, we begin to respect who and what we are through the lessons of herpes. Despite all the responsibilities that herpes puts on us, we begin to see what synchronizing our body and mind can do for our esteem. Forgiveness is a soothing attitude toward yourself that has little to do with condoning inappropriate behavior. It's more like letting go of our own throat, moving us from constricted fear to confidence, peace, and joy.

The Hermes Protocol: starts with telling the truth. Then we begin to open our heart's that fear closed. There is no longer any room for cowards. We shed any hesitation about being honest with ourselves because it feels unpleasant. Cleaning up our past brings us closer to trust, harmony, and happiness. There is no perfection in life, so expect distress and setbacks from time to time. Learn from your mistakes so you can prevent them in the future. Do not take life personally. Remember, no one owes you. Use the lessons of herpes not to be a victim in life, and do not wait for the future or other people to come to your rescue. Live today as if it is your last, because one day it will be. Thank you for allowing me to share my strength, hope, and experience.

Reinhard Hermes.

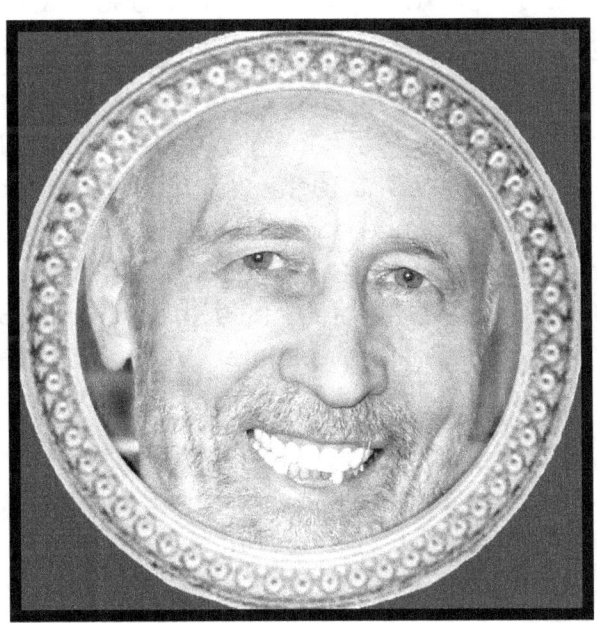

Dedication

I dedicate this book to all our *"friends"* who live with the *"enemy."* While orthodox medicine still has not found a cure for herpes, other than the use of traditional antiviral medications, gains have been made in diagnostics.

It's safe to say that no one likes being diagnosed with Genital Herpes and told to *"take these meds or just learn to live with it."* Today we have another option. By opening this book, you've taken that first alternative step *"to transition from Genital Herpes to the Hermes Protocol, and eventual Herpetic Freedom."* Getting back up after we fall is better than going down and staying out. I'm grateful to be part of that effort and wish you the same success that I experienced.

About the Author

Reinhard Hermes, MS, is a Clinical and Community Psychologist whose experience and education gives him the expertise to write about Genital Herpes. Born in Berlin, Germany, a naturalized U.S. citizen, Reinhard served 4-years in the U.S. Army as a medic in the 46th Medical Battalion, and Emergency Room Technician, at Bad Cannstatt 5th General Hospital, Germany. He received his Master of Science degree from California State University, Fullerton.

An effective and intuitive Community Psychologist and Nutrition Therapist, he worked in tandem with physicians and clients to achieve maximum health outcomes through personalized consultations. His competencies include nutritional intervention, Gerson Cancer Therapy Treatment, and Emotional Freedom Technique. With strong diagnostic skills, Reinhard participated in several internships that include Senior Psychometrist at College of Medicine, University of California, Irvine, CA, and the Gerson Training Institute, Cancer Nutrition, in San Diego, CA.

Reinhard currently resides in New Market, Maryland. Please contact Reinhard via email regarding questions, concerns, or comments. **Thank you** for reading about my experience, resolution, and FREEDOM since 2017 from Genital Herpes, My Friend the Enemy. Be well, Reinhard.

RHermes1@gmail.com

Uniform Resource Locators URLs

Websites: in Genital Herpes

https://covid.cdc.gov/covid-data-tracker/#cases_totalcases

Page x	http://bit.ly/3zMwR2M	3.3 Million Ukrainians Refugees
Page x	http://bit.ly/3MvOD1R	Vaccinated Americans
Page x	http://bit.ly/40V7asJ	Senator Ron Johnson (R-Wis)
Page xi	https://tinyurl.com/2s4k9ys5	COVID Data Tracker Cases
Page xiii	http://bit.ly/2DDAKZ1Depression	WHO Depression Stats
Page xiii	http://bit.ly/2EgXbo2	HSV-2 Depression
Page xiv	RHermes1@gmail.com	
Page 4	http://bit.ly/2rKxVUA	1986 OC Magazine AIDS
Page 5	http://stanford.io/2FoKxT5	HIV/AIDS Hippie Movement
Page 9	http://bit.ly/2nhZrUACDC	Pregnancy and Genital Herpes
Page 11	http://bit.ly/2rIviTIHarvard	Bankruptcy and Medical Expenses
Page 18	http://bit.ly/2GqpgdeABCNews	Angelina Jolie HSV Bell's Palsy
Page 18	http://bit.ly/2Bzi9M1Palsy	Life Extension
Page 18	http://bit.ly/2FogrzmNRC	Dying Younger
Page 21	http://bit.ly/2nINgXdHSV2	Anti-Herpetic Agents
Page 21	http://stanford.io/2FoKxT5	Herpes 460 BC, Hippocrates
Page 22	http://bit.ly/2Gqr59RSTIGMA	Hollywood Stigma
Page 33	http://bit.ly/2DVWCIWiki	*Herpesviridae* DNA Viruses
Page 33	http://bit.ly/2FoogoACDC	CDD and HSV-2
Page 33	http://bit.ly/2DIgSUPHPV	HPV Human Papillomavirus
Page 36	http://bit.ly/2DLTnhG	The London Hospital
Page 36	http://wapo.st/2nIwpTz	Hippie Free Love - Not

Page 37	http://bit.ly/2njUIky	The Dawn of Genital Herpes
Page 38	http://ti.me/2DIh8mA	Time Magazine
Page 38	http://bit.ly/2EjxJ19	Phil Robertson, Duck Dynasty
Page 43	http://bit.ly/2GrkOuM	HIV and HSV Study Comparison
Page 43	http://bit.ly/2nhQKdc	Genital Herpes and Personality
Page 44	http://bit.ly/2DSavBzTIME	Time Magazine: Scarlett Letter
Page 45	http://bit.ly/2FlO1G7	Herpes Stigma
Page 45	http://bit.ly/2DJG8OA	Herpes Stigma: the Origin
Page 46	http://bit.ly/2DGThDD	American Sexual Health Association
Page 47	http://bit.ly/2DFWvYb	David Vetter, Boy in the Bubble
Page 47	http://bit.ly/2rQISVY	Pub Med Herpes Shedding
Page 52	http://bit.ly/2DJI35r	Eczema Herpeticum
Page 52	http://bit.ly/2DJXdnI	Eczema Herpeticum Complications
Page 55	http://bit.ly/2DNAYAM	U.S. Vioxx Cover-Up
Page 61	http://bit.ly/2Gq45rO	Valtrex 1-Year Study
Page 61	http://bit.ly/2ni1gkC	Dietary Supplements for Herpes
Page 62	http://bit.ly/2rHWIZk	Acyclovir Study
Page 62	http://bit.ly/2BAnVNI	Valtrex Study
Page 62	http://bit.ly/2niNQEY	Journal of Infectious Disease
Page 63	http://bit.ly/2DI5YhP	Albert Einstein College of Medicine
Page 64	https://www.clinicaltrials.gov/	
Page 66	www.medscape.com	Antibiotic Associated Adverse Events
Page 67	http://bit.ly/2FqEg9v	**"Death by Medicine"**
Page 67	http://bit.ly/2BzrnrC	**"Death by Medicine"** PDF Download
Page 68	https://bit.ly/3GO6DAO	Distrust in the Medical Profession
Page 68	http://bit.ly/2DM2kaQ	2022 U.S. Health & Welfare Budget

Page 73	http://bit.ly/2FofRl0	Wikipedia U.S. Men's Mortality
Page 73	http://bit.ly/2nhUStG	U.S. Infant Mortality Rate
Page 73	http://bit.ly/2rKx0Uf	Vaccinated Children Get Sicker
Page 75	http://bit.ly/2Bygztz	Chronic Back Pain Research
Page 76	http://bit.ly/2Gqd9wl	Herpes and Cognitive Impairment
Page 76	http://bit.ly/2rHykqE	Mental Impairment and HSV-1
Page 76	http://bit.ly/2EhRupV	Journal of Neuroanatomy
Page 77	http://bit.ly/2Fn6kuz	Herpes Outbreaks Cause Stress
Page 77	http://wb.md/2EiGfgO	Persistent Stress Causes Outbreaks
Page 77	https://www.supportgroups.com/herpes	
Page 78	http://bit.ly/2FrQvmp	Meetup.com Local Get Togethers
Page 79	https://www.petfinder.com	
Page 79	http://bit.ly/2GsMMX4	Social Media and Socially Isolated
Page 79	http://amzn.to/2BBVJcJ	Dr. Wayne Dyer, Spiritual Solution
Page 82	http://bit.ly/2GrkEne	Severe Allergies and Immune System
Page 82	http://bit.ly/2GsVaFN	Too Long to Heal
Page 83	http://wb.md/2DM3l2y	WebMD.com Sixteen Symptoms
Page 83	http://wb.md/2DX7SOK	Autoimmune Disorders
Page 83	https://tgam.ca/2nj3YGj	Immune System and Herpes
Page 85	https://medicineassistancetool.org/	Medicine Assistance Tool
Page 85	https://www.pparx.org/	Partnership for Prescription Assist
Page 85	www.rxassist.org	Pharmaceutical Patient Assistance
Page 85	https://www.rxhope.com/	Drug Assistance Programs
Page 85	http://bit.ly/2DYSMZn	Thyroid Hormone Effect on HSV-1
Page 85	https://stopthethyroidmadness.com/	
Page 85	www.acam.org	American College Advancement Medicine

Page 88	http://bit.ly/2DY1Pts	Adrenal Fatigue Video
Page 88	http://bit.ly/2rJHcfw	Daily Temperature Readings
Page 89	www.celticseasalt.com	Add Minerals into Your Diet
Page 89	http://amzn.to/2FsPhau	Ionic Balanced Trace Minerals
Page 89	http://bit.ly/2BBeEEG	IOM Water recommendation
Page 89	www.aurorahealthandnutrition.com	Hair Tissue Mineral Analysis
Page 89	www.DrLWilson.com	
Page 92	http://cbsn.ws/2EnV1De	Alcohol and Health
Page 95	http://bit.ly/2DSBT2r	Water Fluoridation and Tooth Deca
Page 96	http://bit.ly/2noIOXK	Bromine and Health Issues
Page 96	http://bit.ly/2DYimxy	Processed Food and Early Death
Page 99	http://bit.ly/2DZjQr6	Sugar the New Tobacco
Page 100	http://bit.ly/2BAWTFL	Sugar Coated Trailer
Page 100	http://bit.ly/2DW4MKV	Sugar More Addictive than Cocaine
Page 100	http://bit.ly/2EmBD9x	Sugar Consumption
Page 103	https://bit.ly/3mb6ccN	Candida Overgrowth
Page 103	http://bit.ly/2DJwGGE	Herpes Reduces Immunity
Page 103	http://bit.ly/2DKl9ae	Candida and Herpes
Page 103	https://knowthecause.com/	Herpes or Fungus?
Page 106	http://bit.ly/2Fr2wsa	Exercise and Immunity
Page 108	http://bit.ly/2GrdFdM	Hair Tissue Mineral Analysis (HTMA)
Page 108	www.aurorahealthandnutrition.com	HTMA Kits
Page 108	www.DrLWilson.com	HTMA Kits
Page 109	http://bit.ly/2np6HOT	The Beck Protocol Granada Forum
Page 109	http://bit.ly/2FtMcqJ	Science & Vie Magazine
Page 110	http://bit.ly/2rNygGb	Harvard & MIT and Microcurrents

Page 110	https://bit.ly/3sZAVJS	Sota Instruments
Page 111	www.TheSilverEdge.com	Colloidal Siler Generator
Page 111	www.silvergen.com	Silver Generator
Page 111	https://bit.ly/3Gx1USt	Sota Magnetic Pulser
Page 113	www.silversafety.org	Silver Safety Council Guidelines
Page 114	http://amzn.to/2BBFJI5	Colloidal Silver Reference
Page 115	www.theozonemiracle.com	Dr. Frank Shallenberger, MD
Page 115	www.ozonegenerator.com	Longevity Resources
Page 115	https://aaot.us/	American Academy of Ozone Therapy
Page 117	www.SilverSafety.org	
Page 117	http://bit.ly/2DOz7Ms	Life and Health Research Group
Page 117	http://bit.ly/2noM1pb	Silver Inhibits AIDS Virus
Page 117	www.SilverInstitute.org	
Page 119	http://bit.ly/2nqtSr8	Drug Companies & Silver
Page 119	http://bit.ly/2nqhVl9	Clinical Studies & Colloidal Silver
Page 119	http://bit.ly/2rLG636	Gwyneth Paltrow & Colloidal Silver
Page 119	http://bit.ly/2rNEqpN	Videos Making Colloidal Silver
Page 120	www.joettecalabrese.com	Homeopathy & Colloidal Silver
Page 121	http://bit.ly/2nkDBA2	Brain Detects the Food We Eat
Page 123	http://amzn.to/2rSXUco	Hylands Bioplasma
Page 125	http://bit.ly/2Fv5IIN	DMSO Studies
Page 125	http://bit.ly/2Eembel	DMSO Patient Study Results
Page 126	http://bit.ly/2DLHS5G	DMSO Treatment Results
Page 127	http://bit.ly/2FvUyhv	Vitamin C & Herpes Treatment
Page 127	http://bit.ly/2DNhqZD	Herpes & Vitamin C
Page 127	http://bit.ly/2DWR6iS	Vitamin C, Shingles, and Vaccination

Page 128	http://bit.ly/2DMURYJ	Vitamin C and Cold Sores
Page 128	http://bit.ly/2nIZAXe	Vitamin C with Copper and Herpes
Page 128	http://bit.ly/2EmoVHK	Vitamin C Topical Treatment
Page 129	http://bit.ly/2BF5KGd	Vitamin C to Bowel Tolerance
Page 130	http://bit.ly/2EryXaV	Vitamin C & Viral Hepatitis, Dr. Klenner
Page 131	http://bit.ly/2GxjOVV	Vitamin C and Latest Cancer Research
Page 132	http://bit.ly/2DMpOs0	LDN and Disease Prevention
Page 132	http://bit.ly/2EoosVO	YouTube LDN Video
Page 132	www.LDNscience.org	Low Dose Naltrexone Science
Page 135	http://bit.ly/2DKKalG	Miracle Mineral Solutions (MMS)
Page 136	https://jimhumblebooks.co/	Jim Humble's Website
Page 136	http://bit.ly/2nqNk7b	Life Extension: Death by Medicine
Page 137	http://bit.ly/2Gsx91E	Genesis Church YouTube Acct
Page 138	http://www.wpsuppliers.com	Wager Purification Vendors
Page 139	www.mmsnews.is	MMS Health Recovery Guidebook (Site??)
Page 140	http://bit.ly/2GrP6gW	Jim Humble YouTube (Terminated?)
Page 143	http://bit.ly/2BDISGY	Proteolytic Enzyme Benefits
Page 143	http://bit.ly/2nr4SQv	Proteolytic Enzymes for Immune Health
Page 145	http://cnn.it/2Ftih1J	Vitamin Smoke Screen
Page 145	http://orthomolecular.org/	Ortho Medicine News Service
Page 145	http://bit.ly/2GuC42k	No Deaths from Supplements
Page 147	http://bit.ly/2rRz7FM	Vitamin A Deficiency
Page 147	http://bit.ly/2EpcafF	Key Role in Healing Herpes Infections
Page 147	http://bit.ly/2DMJdci	Vitamin A and Healthy Immune System
Page 148	http://bit.ly/2GuRF1K	View Natural Remedy
Page 148	http://bit.ly/2DLo9Tv	Topical Herpes Healing Formulations

Page 149	http://bit.ly/2rP5ogB Topical Zinc Salts
Page 149	http://bit.ly/2E0hbgM Hans Nieper, MD, Hannover, Germany
Page 150	http://bit.ly/2DPk7tz Zinc DIY Taste Test
Page 150	http://bit.ly/2nrZwEr Selenium Deficiency Flu Virus Mutations
Page 150	http://bit.ly/2DNbvro Selenium Critical for AIDS Patient Survival
Page 150	http://bit.ly/2nmh2en Increases Natural Killer Cells by 82%
Page 151	http://bit.ly/2npiCv2 Thymic Protein and the Immune System
Page 151	http://bit.ly/2nqXQvb Nutrition Review: Thymic Protein
Page 152	www.glucan.us Health Information about Beta-glucans
Page 152	www.TransferPoint.com Beta Glucan 300
Page 152	http://amzn.to/2DO6tLh Other Beta Glucan Options
Page 153	http://bit.ly/2nnQidm Lactoferrin for Prevention of Viral Infections
Page 153	http://bit.ly/2DYBUSi Colostrum Research
Page 154	http://bit.ly/2E31DsW Herpes and Alzheimer's
Page 154	http://bit.ly/2nnyRK3 Lysine and Dementia
Page 155	http://bit.ly/2Eqp5hu *"The Informant"* Movie
Page 155	http://bit.ly/2DQ3GRQ Sheldon Cooper's Lysine
Page 156	http://bit.ly/2DLXudo Wipe Out Herpes with BHT
Page 157	www.EarthClinic.com
Page 157	http://bit.ly/2nr17KQ BHT Hepatitis Treatment
Page 157	www.CoconutResearchCenter.org The Tree of Life
Page 157	http://bit.ly/2E0Vuxj Coconut Oil Miracle: Where is the Evidence
Page 157	http://bit.ly/2FttI9C Dr. Oz for U.S. Senate
Page 158	www.WestonAPrice.org Nutrition and Health
Page 158	www.Lauricidin.com Monolaurin derived from Coconut Oil
Page 160	http://bit.ly/2DO4gvo Garlic and Therapeutic Effects

Page 161	http://bit.ly/2nq9U0j	Garlic Antiviral Effects
Page 161	www.WebMd.com	
Page 163	http://bit.ly/2GzeYHC	ACV and Baking Soda Tonic
Page 165	http://bit.ly/2nv4Mrf	Hydrogen Peroxide Therapy
Page 166	http://bit.ly/2np8nrh	Manuka Honey
Page 167	http://bit.ly/2BHGlf5	Zinc Oxide, Castor Oil Cream
Page 167	www.SilverPure.com	Silver Gel Cream 35,000 ppm
Page 168	www.lauricidin.com	Monolaurin Supplement
Page 169	Infectious Microorganisms	
Page 170	http://bit.ly/2FyTtp0	EFT Tapping, The Science
Page 170	http://bit.ly/2FAmGAf	Emotional Freedom Technique & Herpes
Page 171	http://bit.ly/2nuOjTW	EFT Taping Tutorial
Page 171	http://bit.ly/2E13Wwy	EFT Founder Gary Craig
Page 173	Brad Yates Tap Alongs	Feel Better, Do Better, Get Better
Page 175	http://bit.ly/2E0TEg1	Metabolism and Aging
Page 175	http://bit.ly/2rWA9QS	Healing from the Inside Out
Page 175	http://bit.ly/2BHw6rf	Clearing Negativity
Page 175	www.emofree.com	Gary Craig EFT Training Center
Page 175	http://bit.ly/2DPPluV	EFT Tapping Intro
Page 175	http://bit.ly/2E2FoTJ	EFT and Emotional Balance
Page 175	http://bit.ly/2Fxu2Ep	EFT for Serious Diseases
Page 175	http://bit.ly/2EtTYli	EFT for Pain Relief Nick Ortner
Page 175	http://bit.ly/2nwgOk1	Tapping Peace & Light
Page 175	http://bit.ly/2BHUuJ2	Tapping Releases Shoulder Pain
Page 178	http://bit.ly/2ntTp2E	Mindfulness meditation helpful against pain
Page 179	http://bit.ly/2Ev9OM8	Pema Chodron Talks Mindfulness

Page 182	http://bit.ly/2nv2bgN	Brad Yates Tapping, *"Healing"*
Page 182	Psychiatrist Rick Leskowitz	EFT for PTSD
Page 184	http://bit.ly/2BHXXaD	Eckhart Tolle, You Are Not Your Mind.
Page 184	http://amzn.to/2BBVJcJ	Wayne Dyer, Spiritual Solution
Page 185	http://bit.ly/2rWOH2Q	Nutritional Balancing Dr. Wilson
Page 189	http://bit.ly/2EsxQYi	Proteolytic Enzymes
Page 189	http://bit.ly/2rYGifo	American Thyroid Association (ATA)
Page 190	http://bit.ly/2noTMfO	Benefits of Thyroid Hormone and Herpes
Page 190	https://stopthethyroidmadness.com/	
Page 191	www.acam.org	American College for Advancement in Medicine
Page 191	http://bit.ly/2BJq6hC	Caffeine and Herpes: Good And Bad
Page 192	www.budwigcenter.com	Cancer and Fat Metabolism
Page 192	http://bit.ly/2GBoZnP	Health Dietary Fat
Page 192	http://bit.ly/2EsUG1X	Apple Cider Vinegar Dosage
Page 194	http://bit.ly/2FxldKX	Herpes and Melatonin
Page 194	**_Melatonin_**	by Jeff T Bowles
Page 194	http://amzn.to/2DUmmQg	Other Books by Jeff T Bowles
Page 194	http://wapo.st/2nskCnf	Europe, Melatonin and Birth Control
Page 195	http://bit.ly/2s4Gjyz	LDN for Treatment of Herpes
Page 195	www.LDNScience.org	
Page 196	http://bit.ly/2DRm5K0	The Conscious Mind
Page 197	http://bit.ly/2rYX8e6	Chemicals in Infants
Page 200	www.Gerson.org	
Page 200	http://bit.ly/2BKgsv9	Coffee Enema
Page 208	rhermes1@gmail.com	Email for questions or concerns.

Thank you, *Reinhard Hermes*

www.ingramcontent.com/pod-product-compliance
Lightning Source LLC
Chambersburg PA
CBHW062350220526
45472CB00008B/1757